HIPPOCRATIC
MEDICINE

HIPPOCRATIC MEDICINE

ITS SPIRIT AND METHOD

By
William Arthur Heidel

NEW YORK: MORNINGSIDE HEIGHTS
COLUMBIA UNIVERSITY PRESS
1941

Copyright 1941 by
COLUMBIA UNIVERSITY PRESS, NEW YORK

FOREIGN AGENTS: Oxford University Press, Humphrey Milford, Amen House, London, E. C. 4, England, and B. I. Building, Nicol Road, Bombay, India; Maruzen Company, Ltd., 6 Nihonbashi, Tori-Nichome, Tokyo, Japan

MANUFACTURED IN THE UNITED STATES OF AMERICA

FOREWORD

IN HIS *History of the Inductive Sciences*,[1] William Whewell spoke of the great thinkers of early Greece as representing the heroic age of science, having in mind the boldness of their adventures on the uncharted vastness of human thought and also the colossal stature they have attained in historical perspective. Professor Heidel gave a lifetime of interest and labor to the study of that period, and his book *The Heroic Age of Science*[2] presented a vivid story of the ideas which took wing in that unique epoch of man's early struggle for knowledge. In stating the purpose of this book he said: "It is to indicate how the Greeks set about the task of laying the foundations of science, rather than to recount their achievements."

Professor Heidel, after his retirement, had in mind the preparation of a large work on Greek science, and in response to the invitation of the Josiah Macy, Jr. Foundation he chose Hippocratic medicine as a special field in which to reveal the influence of Greek science. Just as he finished the manuscript of this volume, his voice was stilled and his lifework ended. It is indeed fortunate that he was able to complete this piece of work. But to his friends and admirers and to scholars generally it will be

[1] D. Appleton Company (2 vols., New York, 1866).
[2] Carnegie Institution (Washington, D. C., 1933).

a source of deep regret that he could not live to carry out the larger enterprise of which this study was but one small part. No one was better fitted by scholarly knowledge and ripened judgment for such a task.

One cannot read this book without being impressed by the author's scholarly, patient, and penetrating way of reconstructing the growth and meaning of knowledge in the fifth and fourth centuries B.C., or without realizing his sensitive interpretations of the intentions of Greek thinkers who are represented by so little of their original writings. It is not only the historian but also the philosopher and the scientist who unfolds the picture of Hippocratic medicine in an epoch in which philosophy and science were one and the problem of health—of healing and of wholeness—was one of the central themes of the great discourse. Today it is assumed that medicine, science, philosophy, and history are more or less separate, and to many it seems essential that they should be so. This book on the origin of science and medicine may, however, serve a good purpose by showing how inseparably intertwined are science and philosophy, philosophy and history, and science and medicine. Professor Heidel has shown how much empirical information the Greeks had collected, how much originality went into their endeavors to bring some order into their observations, and how intelligently they tried to link their medical knowledge with their philosophic efforts to understand the universe.

If thirst for information, intelligence, and imagination are the essential ingredients of scientific thinking, the Greeks certainly were striving to be scientific. Our age has added insistence upon verification of observations, of judgments, and of hypotheses and has thus made the experimental method the great tool of modern science.

We must, of course, realize how comparatively incomplete their knowledge was: biochemistry, microbiology, and cellular pathology were unknown; anatomy and physiology were just beginning; the Greeks had no microscope or X ray. Yet their intelligence was skillfully applied, and their imagination soared to such heights that for twenty-five hundred years the great Greek thinkers have remained a unique group in the history of thought.

The so-called "Hippocratic writings," as Professor Heidel points out in this book, were actually by various men of different historical periods; this explains why, upon first reading, much of their value is obscured by many irrelevant and immature sayings. When careful attention is given to them, however, a surprising system of interpretations, having considerable bearing upon our way of thinking, becomes evident. The Greeks made a clear distinction between the man who used knowledge for practical skill only and the man who "knew the reasons for his action," for the latter was also a philosopher. It was also their conception that to treat his patient effectively the physician has to understand him as a whole and as a part of the world in which he lives. Aristotle said that the best physicians devote themselves earnestly to the study of the body; that the human constitution, whatever its composition, is ultimately the same as that of all other things; hence, in order to know what man is, one must know the nature of the world, since the laws of human existence are in reality only special forms of universal laws.

That the Greeks were occupied primarily with the physical aspects of the environment is easily understood as reflecting the preoccupation of the philosophers of the time. Today we know that, while man is governed by laws, "in reality only special forms of universal laws," individually he is also a unique manifestation of his heredity and of his special life history. From the earliest experiences of childhood to those of the latest period of life, man expresses the sum total of his own existence. What this signifies for his education and for his health the modern physician-philosopher will have to answer.

It would be an exaggeration to say the Greeks created a lasting system of medicine in theory or practice, but they did raise ultimate questions and did show how to go about solving them. It is not the problems they solved that gave value to that "golden age" but rather the questions they raised—some of which have not been answered in the intervening twenty-five hundred years. It is the spirit in which they proposed to solve them which gave that period its distinction; as Professor Heidel says: "The aim of the Hippocratics was to make medicine thoroughly scientific."

Some of the great questions raised by the Greek sages —questions which are still acute—are concerned with the place of man in the universe in which he exists and of which he is a part; with the relation of mind to body; and with the relation of physician to patient. These are persistent problems that each generation must face in terms of the understanding and insight with which it attempts to order its experience and to direct its life. Such questions are especially urgent today because so many of the answers proposed at earlier times have become inadequate and unacceptable to the scientific understanding and enlightened insight of our day. They are, moreover, especially urgent today when we are seeking a new theory of medicine and attempting to define the role and responsibility of medicine as a social instrument.

The world of man has changed since Socrates, Plato, Hippocrates, and Aristotle discussed these problems; science has transformed our environment, our universities, our hospitals, and many of our ideas. Yet if those thinkers could join us today (as they almost seem to do through the magic of Professor Heidel, a historian at home in both ages), they could, if they knew our forms of speech, converse with our contemporary thinkers. Perhaps in imagining such a discourse we may understand the essential contribution the Greeks made, namely, how to use intelligence. The history of science is but a continuation of the questioning, which the Greeks initiated, of the wisdom of the past. We must acknowledge the great importance of the beginning made by the Greeks when they showed that a certain way of thinking (which we call science) is the best way in the "quest of certainty."

There is abundant evidence that the good physicians in the Hippocratic age insisted upon a discipline of mind before they applied their skill in the art of healing. In this sense they were the first scientific physicians. Note the admonition to the practitioner to ascertain as much information as possible and to put all together "so that a single likeness may result from the differing symptoms."

What does that mean other than to urge him to make a diagnosis—to seek an explanation that implies some order and unity in thought—for there are order and unity in the organism even when it is in disturbed health?

One of the greatest handicaps for Greek thinkers was the fact that the idea of evolution, although dimly caught by some, did not enter into their system of thought; their natural philosophy was static. Different species of animals existed, for them, as unchangeable. There was no need to inquire into origin or into relationship to environment except in the effect upon the individual organism. The idea of the evolutionist, who explains the continuous process of changes through generations as mutations and as the result of determining environmental factors, did not exist. In spite of their recognition of the "scale of living things," it left them helpless in any attempt to conceive a history of life through changing forms as a continuity of life from the inorganic to the organic, from lower to higher specifications. And though they dwelt on the idea that "all is flux" and believed that man was part of the cosmos, such beliefs had no content in terms of evolution and remained, at least in theory, largely sterile. In practical therapeutics the Hippocratics were well aware of the changes of individual life in health and sickness caused by environment, and they perceived tendencies transmitted by parents to their children.

Our present phase in the progress of medical thought makes Professor Heidel's book particularly interesting and appropriate. Medicine today has an immense wealth of new knowledge waiting to be ordered into a coherent system, where parts of the whole and the whole of the parts of the living organism find their meaning in a valid theory. For such a theoretical structure we must utilize concepts that will bring experimental results and clinical observations into a unified frame of reference congruous with the more recent ideas of the physical and biological sciences. Thus the physician and medical scientist are faced with the same situation that confronted Hippocrates and his contemporaries when they boldly projected a theory of medicine in terms of the contemporary explorations into the nature of the cosmos and man's relation thereto. Perhaps this account of what they did may serve to recall medicine to its historic task of focusing all knowledge upon the vital problem of man's welfare. Meanwhile our practitioners face problems and tasks which cannot wait for future knowledge; decisions and actions must be taken this day, this hour. Our practitioners must draw also upon a wisdom born of their experience and intuition, and they still must be guided by the Greek saying "art is long and time is fleeting."

LUDWIG KAST

New York
June, 1941

PREFACE

FEW NAMES are held in higher honor than that of Hippocrates, though there is little that is positively known about him. And yet the world has good reason to cherish his name; the testimony of Plato and Aristotle to his greatness should suffice to justify the honor paid to the "Father of Medicine," even though that title may not rightly belong to him.

Though Hippocrates did not originate Greek, and therefore scientific, medicine, he was clearly the preëminent representative of that art in the fifth century B.C., when medicine first displays for us the marks that characterize it today. If we cannot distinguish his personal traits, we can envisage him as the typical physician of his day. In attempting to do so we may claim to be following the example of his contemporaries; for, in portraiture, contemporary Greek sculptors rarely, if ever, attempted to present personal lineaments but rather created or reproduced a type.

This discussion aims to interest the physician; it seeks to solve no problem of literary or historical research, such as the "Hippocratic question." Controversy is avoided altogether, even where strong conviction would seem to justify it. Many special topics that have interested the writer have been left unmentioned because a discussion of them would perforce have been either so sketchy as to be valueless or so long as to be inappropriate in the context.

The account of Hippocratic medicine herewith offered is governed by considerations such as these. This account does not aim at completeness, since it practically ignores surgery, in which Greek physicians achieved perhaps their greatest triumphs. It is concerned chiefly with the spirit and methods of that medical fraternity whose members can be regarded as participants in the scientific endeavors of the time. How much these members gave and how much they merely received we cannot tell; for often the physician was a "philosopher" also, and in any case there was happily as yet no hard and fast distinction between pure and applied science. The wide-awake physician was a man of science who employed his skill and knowledge in the service of suffering humanity; if by experiment and experience he could advance general science, he would gladly do so.

One would like to know how successful the Hippocratic physician was in practice. Unfortunately, one has no means of judging, either absolutely or by comparison with his present-day successor. It is, however, significant that Plato and Aristotle obviously held the better doctors in high esteem. The Hippocratic treatise *Ancient Medicine* recognizes that some doctors are good and some are bad but adds that we all have recourse to them when an emergency arises. Perhaps as good a testimonial as any to their general efficiency is to be found in the words of Diogenes the Cynic, who scoffed at most men:

PREFACE

When he saw physicians, philosophers, and pilots at their work he deemed man the most intelligent of all animals; but when he saw interpreters of dreams and diviners and those who attended to them, or those who were puffed up with conceit of wealth, he thought no animal more silly.

The Pythagorean also, says Iamblichus, regarded the art of medicine as the highest human wisdom.

It is a privilege to record my sincere thanks for their assistance and helpful coöperation to the Josiah Macy, Jr. Foundation through its president, Dr. Ludwig Kast, and other officers and to Dr. John Dewey, teacher and friend through many years, but for whose interest this book would hardly have been written.

The notes serve chiefly to refer the reader to sources. The so-called "Hippocratic treatises" are cited according to the edition of Émile Littré, *Œuvres complètes d'Hippocrate* (10 vols., Paris, 1839–61); the earlier philosophers, according to Hermann Diels, *Die Fragmente der Vorsokratiker* (5th ed., Berlin, 1934–37); Diocles, according to Max Wellmann, *Fragmentsammlung der griechischen Aerzte* (Vol. I, Berlin, 1901); Plato, by the pages of the edition of Stephanus; and Aristotle, by the pages of the Berlin Academy edition.

WILLIAM ARTHUR HEIDEL

Middletown, Connecticut
January, 1941

CONTENTS

FOREWORD, BY LUDWIG KAST	v
I. INTRODUCTION	1
II. THE IDEAL OF SCIENCE	8
III. THE SCIENCE OF THE TIME	15
IV. THE MEDICAL PROFESSION	26
V. SOME SCIENTISTS OF THE DAY	40
VI. SCIENTIFIC METHODS	57
VII. MEDICINE AS AN ART	117
VIII. CONCLUSION	137
INDEX	141

I

INTRODUCTION

THE NAME of Hippocrates is invested with a halo not unlike that of certain other great characters, such as Pythagoras and Socrates, and he has sometimes been invoked almost as if he were a saint. Indeed, in the Middle Ages he was actually grouped with the Christian saints of healing, Cosmas and Damian. This is partly due to the rank growth of legend which commonly springs up around a potent personality and which, in the case of Hippocrates, in time so far transfigured the historical character that it is now impossible to distinguish his actual features or the true story of his life. One must not think this result singular or question the fact of his having lived, for such was the fate (except for those who took an active part in public affairs) of most men of his time who attained sufficient prominence to redeem their memory from oblivion. Even of statesmen we usually know for certain only what of good or harm they did to the state, while their private lives are depicted for us in anecdotes—anecdotes the authenticity of which is rarely above suspicion. Of the life of Hippocrates we actually know little more than nothing. He was an Asclepiad of the island of Cos, and he was regarded as the outstanding representative of the Coan school of medicine, which flourished in honorable rivalry with the neighboring school of Cnidus. Whether the appellative "Asclepiad," as applied to him, vouches for his descent from a family that traced its lineage to the god Asclepius or assures us only that he, as well as his immediate ancestors, belonged to an ancient medical guild, we do not know. He lived in the fifth and fourth centuries B.C., but we cannot be sure about the precise dates of his birth (given as 460) and death (variously given).

If the preoccupation of his Greek contemporaries with the living present and their consequent incuriosity regarding the past led, on the one hand, to the immediate neglect of data that might have been readily verified and, on the other, to the proliferation of legend and fiction later on—leaving the details of his life in doubt—the uncertainties surrounding his doctrine and his achievements in the field of medicine (a far more serious matter) are in part due to other causes. Of his medical views we shall have more to say presently; for the moment we are concerned with the reasons for the hesitation of scholars to attribute any particular doctrine to the great Hippocrates. At first blush such an attitude appears paradoxical, because the ancients, whom one might suppose far better circumstanced than we are for rendering judgment, display no hesitation. It gives one pause, however, when one considers the particular views they present of him. It is disconcerting to find Hippocrates claimed and invoked by nearly all the leading schools of medicine of later times, however much they differed among themselves—for example, by Dogmatics, Empirics, and Skeptics and finally by Galen, who endeavored to sum up in his own teaching all that was good in the thought of his predecessors. In a sense this is not unexampled, for Socrates, too, was the acknowledged master not only of Plato but also of the Cynic Antisthenes and the Hedonist Aristippus of Cyrene. Jesus, also, has been invoked by men of many minds and irreconcilable ideals. While in each such case we are dealing with a "name that is above any other name"—a testimonial of great significance—there is an important difference that calls for remark. Socrates and Jesus impressed their contemporaries (and, through these contemporaries, succeeding generations) by their characters and by their oral teachings—teachings ethical and religious and capable of varying interpretations and applications. So far as we are informed, they did not commit their views of life to writing, and in any case their teaching was general and tentative rather than in the manner of the doctrinaire. Hippocrates, however, if he wrote at all, must have done so as a physician; and as such, if he deserves the high regard in which he has ever been held, he must have had definite views on theory and practice that, set down in writing, would seem to preclude divergencies as great as those one finds in the record.

Here, then, one is confronted with a difficulty that has puzzled, and still puzzles, scholars. On the one hand there are definite statements regarding views of Hippocrates (not only by representatives of later medical schools but also by Plato, who was his younger contemporary) which can hardly be understood except as vouched for by writings accepted as authentic. We are, therefore, bound to assume that Hippocrates was not only a practicing physician but that he left writings in which at least some of his views were set forth. On the other hand, there are preserved a very large number of treatises given in the manuscripts as works of Hippocrates, none of which can with certainty be identified as that to which Plato referred; and, moreover, the treatises are of so varied a character and differ so widely in particular views that it is impossible to regard them as from the pen of the same author. The fact, above mentioned, that representatives of widely different medical schools claimed Hippocrates as their master, is in part explained by the differences among the treatises attributed to him; for if these works were all thought to be genuine, chapter and verse could indeed be cited to verify their various claims. Unfortunately, the tradition is confused and contradictory, as one plainly sees, for example, by the statements of Galen, who, while dogmatically attributing certain works to Hippocrates and denying the authenticity of others on the basis of a preconceived notion of true Hippocratic doctrine, reveals the fact that others did not share his opinion. Reluctantly one resigns oneself to the conclusion that there exists at present no criterion by which one may distinguish between what may and what may not be accepted as Hippocratic in the personal sense. For us Hippocrates must therefore stand for a period in the development of medical theory and practice in which he undoubtedly bore a leading part. That period may be defined as extending from the middle of the fifth to the latter part of the fourth century B.C., or, roughly, from Empedocles to Aristotle. For the documentation of that stage of medical thought—which we may with reason call Hippocratic—we can draw upon all the writings of the period, including all the treatises traditionally attributed to Hippocrates, because there is no good reason for thinking that any of them, with the possible exception of two, dates from later times.

Although it may be thought arbitrary to speak of the medicine of this entire period as Hippocratic, there is sufficient justification for doing so. It is true that Hippocrates is not the only physician whose name has been handed down as prominent in that great age, and it is likewise true that the literary remains are so different that even those which have been claimed for him cannot have been written by the same man. One need not be a pedant in order to recognize these facts and to be aware that the fifth and fourth centuries B.C. were a time of extraordinary literary activity in the field of medicine. Socrates remarked to Euthydemus that medical works were very numerous.[1] If we cannot identify a single extant treatise in the Hippocratic corpus as certainly written by Hippocrates, we cannot with certainty attribute any one of them to any other author. And concerning the writers from whose works well-authenticated extracts have been preserved, it is fair to say that, except for those who stand close to Aristotle, differences between their distinctive doctrines are trivial in comparison with the points of view common to all. Littré was clearly right in asserting that the more closely one studies the Hippocratic treatises the more one recognizes that they all present a level of knowl-

[1] Xenophon, *Memorabilia*, IV, ii, 10.

edge almost the same and conceptions of the living body and its diseases very much alike.²

One may safely go farther and say the same regarding the entire body of literature we here accept as Hippocratic. In his studies of the relation of Plato and Aristotle to the Hippocratic corpus, Poschenrieder long ago made this clear, even though in some respects he claimed too much.³ The differences in detail are not without significance and for certain purposes need to be noted and emphasized; but they are not greater than those to be observed among contemporary physicians of any age who have the same background. Medicine at any time reflects the current scientific outlook; indeed, medicine is neither more nor less than the science of the day applied to the problems of health and disease. Though science is ideally and by intention one, those who promote it and those who apply it inevitably differ among themselves in special aptitudes and interests. In order to obtain a true perspective one must minimize these divergencies and endeavor to grasp the principles that express themselves in theory and practice. Because of the ravages of time (which has dealt unkindly with the works of famous individuals), it happens that the scientific background of the thought of the fifth and early fourth centuries B.C., as well as the medical theories and practices of the time, are now most fully represented by the works attributed by uncertain tradition to Hippocrates. Therefore, without committing one-

² *Œuvres complètes d'Hippocrate*, VIII, 554.
³ *Die Platonischen Dialoge in ihrem Verhältnis zu den Hippokratischen Schriften* (Metten, 1882) and *Die wissenschaftlichen Schriften des Aristoteles in ihrem Verhältnis zu den Büchern der Hippokratischen Sammlung* (Bamberg, 1887).

self to unverifiable judgments concerning the authorship of this body of literature, one may not inappropriately call Hippocratic the general view this literature presents, especially since there is every reason to believe that it was shared by Hippocrates himself.

II

THE IDEAL OF SCIENCE

WE CANNOT with certainty assign any of the extant medical treatises to Hippocrates himself, and his doctrine is subject to the same uncertainty. So much must be conceded to modern criticism. Nevertheless, we are not to conclude that he must remain for us one of the unknown great. However much scope we may allow to skepticism, we have sufficient indisputable evidence to enable us to define his attitude and the method he approved.

Plato, as we have said, was a younger contemporary, and we should be certain that he had knowledge of Hippocrates even if he had not named the physician in the striking passage to which we shall presently turn. In view of Plato's prevailing mood, one would not expect him to display unusual interest in medicine as it is usually practiced. Indeed, in the *Republic*, when he sketches the growth of a city from the simplest beginnings, he remarks that with the prevalence of license and loose living there inevitably arises a marked demand for doctors and lawyers;[1] and

---

[1] 405d ff. John Dryden echoed his words ("To My Honoured Kinsman, John Driden," ll. 71–74):
    So lived our sires ere doctors learned to kill
    And multiply with theirs the weekly bill.
    The first physicians by debauch were made:
    Excess began, and sloth sustains the trade.

THE IDEAL OF SCIENCE

again he speaks with scorn of that practice of Herodicus of Selymbria which encouraged an impotent valetudinarianism.[2] Plato has, therefore, absurdly been dubbed the foe of medicine. If he was such, he was so only in the sense that every idealist contemns the sordid aspects of life. Leaving out of account his prose hymn to creation, *Timaeus,* in which he borrowed copiously from a representative of the Sicilian school of medicine, what Plato elsewhere says about medicine reveals understanding and appreciation of it as an art to which, as a Hippocratic writer says, all men (at least all men of sense) resort in an emergency. Indeed, he treated it with marked respect as a representative expression of reason in practice. Particularly noteworthy is the fact that everything he says about medicine accords perfectly with what we find in the Hippocratic literature. He tells us that the physician inquires about the ailment, beginning with its onset and following its natural course, that the physician talks with the patient and with the patient's friends, and that in this manner the doctor learns from the sufferer while he gives him instructions; he attempts to effect a cure only when by persuasion he has won his patient to willing coöperation.[3] "Good physicians say you cannot heal the eyes unless you cure the head."[4] Every doctor and artisan does whatever he does for the sake of the whole and bestows most care on the improvement of the part that most conduces to the good of the whole—the concern is always of the whole rather than of the part.[5] He contrasts

[2] *Republic,* 409.   [3] *Laws,* 720d.
[4] *Charmides,* 156b ff. Cf. Diocles, frag. 88, Wellmann.
[5] *Laws,* 903c.

10   THE IDEAL OF SCIENCE

the arts of flattery (whether of the palate or of the ear) with medicine, declaring them to be a mere empiric result of practice, ignorant of the nature of the things they offer and, hence, ignorant of the cause that produces the effect. The arts of flattery are not true arts, because no rational account of what they do can be given, whereas medicine controls the body by knowing what food and drink are good or bad for it.[6] Medicine, to be sure, like husbandry, seamanship, and generalship, is not an exact science, able to be defined in everything by number and measure;[7] yet Plato was well aware of the ideal to which medicine aspired. One cannot doubt that he knew physicians of lofty ideals and far-reaching ambition who strove to make their art a true science.

It is against the background of this conception of medicine and of the true physician that we must view the mental picture of Hippocrates evoked in the intelligent reader by the discussion in Plato's *Phaedrus*[8] where Socrates and Phaedrus consider the nature and function of rhetoric. Socrates begins by remarking that Pericles was the most perfect orator and that all great arts demand high and subtle discussion and philosophical speculation about nature. Pericles, we are told, acquired his lofty thoughtfulness by steady intercourse with Anaxagoras and became imbued with that speculation concerning the nature of reason and unreason which Anaxagoras most frequently discussed. The insight he thus acquired he applied to public speaking. The procedure in medicine is

[6] *Gorgias*, 465a and 517e f. Cf. *Phaedrus*, 270d ff., and Aristotle, *De partibus animalium*, 639b.
[7] Plato, *Philebus*, 56a-b. Cf. *De sterilibus mulieribus*, ccxxx (VIII, 442 f., Littré).   [8] 269e ff.

THE IDEAL OF SCIENCE

much the same as in public speaking: one must begin by analyzing nature (in medicine, the nature of the body; in rhetoric, the nature of the soul or mind) if one is to apply, according to the rules of art, food or medicaments for health and strength in the one case or persuasion leading to virtue and law-abiding habits in the other. But one cannot know the nature of the soul or mind without knowing universal nature. At this point Phaedrus interjects the comment that, according to Hippocrates, it is equally true that one cannot know the nature of the body without knowing universal nature. Socrates commends this saying but adds that one must not be content with the authority of Hippocrates but must consider whether true reason agrees with his dictum. The principle enunciated implies that in order to know the nature of a thing one must first inquire whether it is simple or composed of many parts and that in either case one must ascertain the power and effect of the whole (or, if it be composite, of each part) that enables it to act or to be affected in a particular way. Unless one proceeds in this fashion one's way would be like that of the blind. The orator, if he proceeds in the manner of a rational art, must know the nature of the mind or soul as that which he addresses; he must likewise understand his auditors and perceive why one will and another will not be favorably affected by his arguments.[9] (Obviously, this is suggested by an analogy: the good physician can quickly discern the character of his patient's illness and perceive the kind of

---

[9] Cf. *De victu*, I, ii (VI, 468, Littré): "I say that one who is to write properly about human regimen must first of all know and distinguish the constitution of man—know of what elements he is originally

treatment to which it will respond.[10]) Furthermore, the orator must recognize the "appropriate"—and here Plato resorts to a technical term (καιρός) with interesting connotations in Hippocratic literature, for, besides its usual meaning of "opportune moment," the word is sometimes used in the sense of "proper measure," neither too little nor too much.[11]

To the casual reader this passage may seem to tell us little about Hippocrates, who seems at first blush to be mentioned almost by accident in a remark incidentally thrown in by Socrates' interlocutor. But he who knows Plato's method recognizes that, far from being accidental, the introduction of Hippocrates' name has important significance; his name typifies that rational procedure in the field of medicine which Socrates demands in the theory and practice of oratory. The definite statement that the art of medicine and the art of oratory are approximately the same is the key to the whole discussion; and though it is not expressly stated that Hippocrates and reason are in full accord, one is left with the distinct impression that to the mind of Socrates (Plato) they are. It will, therefore, repay one to consider the episode as the whole it obviously is. It begins, appropriately, with the reference to Pericles as the perfect orator and then proceeds with

---

constituted and by which of the constituent elements he is dominated." This obviously refers to the generic composition of the race and the specific constitution of the individual. Farther on, the same treatise discusses the composition of different souls.

[10] Socrates' requirement is, in fact, exactly parallel to that of Hippocrates. See *De prisca medicina*, xx (I, 620 ff., Littré). See also *De arte*, xii (VI, 24, Littré).

[11] *De morbis*, IV, li (VII, 584, Littré). A similar use of the word occurs in *De locis in homine*, xliv (VI, 338, Littré).

the suggestion that, like all great arts, that of the orator requires, in addition to native endowment, habitual reflection on high themes—just as Pericles was led by association with Anaxagoras to discourse on the subjects of natural philosophy then currently debated. The themes of reason and unreason that Anaxagoras discussed were not psychological, but the discussion related to reason as a cosmic force, though the cosmic reason was of course suggested by reason as a governing factor in life. Such discussions would inevitably lead to the question whether the effects of reason could be traced, in nature, in the parts as well as in the whole. Also, there were those who thought to find evidence of teleology in Anaxagoras, even though Plato and Aristotle complained that he employed reason solely as a cosmic agent. This introductory statement regarding Pericles and Anaxagoras has indisputable bearing on Hippocrates not only because such lofty contemplation is asserted to be a requisite of all great arts, among which must be reckoned the medical art of Hippocrates, but especially because he is expressly cited as holding that one cannot know the nature of the body without knowing universal nature. In the context this statement makes sense only if we assume that Plato meant to represent Hippocrates as a physician who took the large view—the view that medicine is to be regarded as a special application of general science, that medicine is the science of the human body as a part of the universe, and that the body is subject to the laws of the universe and is composed of elements (each having its specific character and reactions) common to the body itself and to the world at large.

So much one is clearly entitled to infer from this memorable passage. It is enough to delineate the physician whom Aristotle,[12] like his master, regarded as great, and whom the world has justly accepted at their valuation. However gratifying we may find this characterization, we must note that it does not enable us to reconstruct the doctrine of Hippocrates in detail, much less to identify any particular treatise as written by him or as reproducing his personal views. For example, the fact that he regarded the human body as composed of elements common to it and the world at large gives us no indication how he named and defined these elements, whether he sketched a cosmology (as several Hippocratic works do) or contented himself merely with stating the obvious fact ("dust to dust") that, since our bodies grow by accretion from without and in the end render nature her due, we are transient parts of the whole but possess individual qualities and powers as organisms whose organs and parts in turn display, despite their generic similarity, individual reactions. In the voluminous literature we have received as Hippocratic, almost every possible variation on this general theme may be found. Yet in the fundamental point of view there is so much agreement with, and so clear a similarity to, the picture sketched by Plato that, since we are unable to assign these works to any other writer or writers, we may *faute de mieux* call the conception of medicine they present Hippocratic.

[12] *Politics*, 1326a.

III

THE SCIENCE OF THE TIME

IT IS IDLE to inquire into the origin of science and philosophy without defining the terms, and for our purposes definitions are hardly necessary. To avoid ambiguity and misunderstanding one would have to redefine the terms for every age, almost for every generation. It will suffice for the present to say that science is concerned with understanding the part and the proximate, while philosophy looks to the ultimate and the whole. Man being such as he is, his interest extends to both, though individual men will inevitably differ, some laying the emphasis on the whole and seeking to comprehend it as throwing light on the multifarious facts of experience, while others scrutinize the parts in the hope, more or less clearly defined, of somehow and sometime coördinating them in an intelligible system.

The sixth and fifth centuries B.C. were, however, in Greek lands, a period of extraordinary awakening of intellectual interest in the world; and at such times (for example, during the Renaissance in Italy) the curiosity and endeavor of leading minds cannot be confined within narrow limits. We are astonished at the scope of their interest and the range of their achievements. Even though philosophy and science are to be distinguished, they are apt to be united in the same persons. In regard to science, also, there were already developing special interests that were to lead, in time, to the creation of separate sciences; but, as pursued, science was still essentially one. It is sometimes said that at first Greek science (or philosophy) was concerned almost exclusively with the phenomena of the heavens, and various ancient texts are quoted to support this view. We may dismiss the matter by saying that what we know of the earliest Greek thinkers, whether we call them philosophers or men of science, does not bear out the conclusion, which seems, rather, to rest upon those theories of Plato and Aristotle that touch on the origin of the belief in God.[1]

From the earliest times, the interest of the Greeks extended equally to the phenomena of the heavens and to those of living beings, especially of man. A surgeon general of the German army contended that Homer must have been a physician and surgeon. The suggestion is bizarre only because it is expressed in terms of an age of specialization. In the time of Homer and much later, as in the Middle Ages, men of intelligence and education might, in a fashion, cover the entire field of knowledge. Even then, however, there were men who were outstanding in medicine and surgery. The earliest "philosopher" of whom we have definite information, Anaximander, was equally interested in the origin of the world and of man and had, besides, the temerity to project maps of the

[1] The theory that religion grew out of fear of meteorological and celestial phenomena is, of course, still older. See Critias frag. 25 Diels

heavens and of the earth. I have elsewhere[2] tried to show that, following the lead of Hesiod in verse, he even made a first essay in prose to treat the sister sciences of history and geography. In any case, from the middle of the sixth century onward, until specialization began to establish itself in the encyclopedic school of Aristotle, men of science, whatever their individual predilections, were by intention concerned with the whole range of science. If proof of this fact were needed, it would suffice to call attention to the scope of Theophrastus' account of the opinions of the natural philosophers and to the subjects included in Plato's *Timaeus*,[3] for the latter is obviously conceived as a treatise on nature and carries on the tradition begun by the Ionians.

Obviously, this general statement applies to the men of the medical profession in their relation to philosophy and general science. If one reviews the data regarding the philosophers of the fifth century, one finds that many of them are expressly described as physicians; and, if one examines their views, one discovers that no inconsiderable part of their thought concerned, or was suggested by, physiological processes. On the other hand, the medical fraternity could not so far renounce its natural allegiance to the republic of sciences as to ignore the ties that bound it to its fellows who were engaged in the study of nature as a whole. Indeed, it is just because of this intimate connection between medicine and natural philosophy that the Hippocratic writings are of so extraordinary value to

[2] "Anaximander's Book, the Earliest Known Geographical Treatise," *Proceedings of the American Academy of Arts and Sciences*, Vol. LVI, No. 7 (1921).
[3] See especially 41a ff.

the student of ancient science and philosophy; for without them the fragmentary record of the philosophers known to us by name would scarcely be intelligible at all. Most histories of early Greek thought are actually misleading because their authors have preferred to interpret detached statements of thinkers of the fifth century B.C. by the thought of twenty-five centuries later instead of reading them in the light of the context supplied by contemporaries.

Medicine, whether regarded as an art or as a science, is inevitably the product of the thought of the age; and Hippocratic medicine, in particular, reflects and shares the virtues and limitations of contemporary science. We are not now concerned with the cosmological theories of the early Greek philosophers, but it is not without interest to note that several of the Hippocratic writings allude to such views and even give brief sketches of natural philosophy.[4] It is generally idle to attempt to assign the views there set forth to individual philosophers or even to date precisely the works containing them, because they express the thought of unknown individuals who took for their own uses what suited them from what was, in fact, a common store of theory or knowledge. In only a few cases is the dependence of the writer upon a known thinker so obvious that one can point it out with assurance. On the other hand, despite the differences in detail, there is the strongest evidence of a common level of knowledge and a common point of view revealed in this mass of literature.

[4] See my "Περὶ Φύσεως: a Study of the Conception of Nature among the Pre-Socratics," *Proceedings of the American Academy of Arts and Sciences*, Vol. XLV, No. 4 (1910), pp. 110 f. and 123, and Rodolfo Mondolfo, *Problemi del pensiero antico* (Bologna, 1936), pp. 78 f.

One of the questions that occupied the minds of the men of science then, as it does today, was what are things made of? Various answers were given, and among the medical fraternity there were some who adopted the view of one or the other philosopher, while others either expressly rejected the theories and tried to rely only on observation or modified such theories to suit the subject matter with which they were dealing. Thus one writer, whom Aristotle, or his pupil Menon, actually identified as Hippocrates himself,[5] adopted the theory proposed by Anaximenes in the sixth century and applied to medicine by Diogenes of Apollonia in the fifth, to wit, that air was the source of all things and in particular the cause of all diseases. Others accepted the four elements of Empedocles—fire, air, water, and earth—but regarded them essentially as characterized by their qualities: fire by heat and dryness, air by heat and moisture, water by cold and moisture, and earth by cold and dryness.[6]

Even when such schemes were expressly rejected and medicine was asserted to be able to dispense with them, the question itself could not be evaded; for man was known to be composed of the same substances as the world, and a bold thinker could challenge the philosophers with the statement that if they would know the nature of things they must resort to human physiology, because their supposed elements and qualities were not to be found separate and unmixed but only in all sorts of com-

---

[5] Referring to the treatise *De flatibus*.
[6] *De victu*, I, vi (VI, 474, Littré), assigns to fire the qualities hot and dry; to water, cold and wet. *De carnibus*, ii (VIII, 584, Littré), gives the qualities as stated above to all four elements, agreeing wholly with Aristotle. See Galen, X, 462, Kühn.

binations.[7] Whether the writer was fully aware of it or not, he put his finger on the weakest spot of Greek science —its failure to realize and appreciate the infinite complexity of things that were assumed to be simple. One writer[8] goes so far as to assert that all diseases are really the same, differing only in respect to the part of the body they specially affect. Science is always faced with the paradox that, while it endeavors to simplify the facts of experience and unify its findings in a single formula, its actual progress seems to lead continually to greater and greater differentiation.

In justice to the early Greeks it must be said, however, that they were not wholly unaware of the complexity of things; for, though they accepted fire, air, water, and earth as elements, they distinguished between kinds of fire and knew that airs were very different, that waters varied in weight and wholesomeness, and that earths were far from being all alike.[9] Celsus,[10] who thought that scientific medicine was relatively late in developing and owed much to philosophers, such as Pythagoras, Empedocles, and Democritus, says that it was at first regarded as a branch of philosophy, insomuch that the cure of diseases and the investigation of nature were fathered by the selfsame writers; Hippocrates, however, he adds, was the

[7] *De prisca medicina,* xv (I, 604 f., Littré).
[8] *De flatibus,* ii (VI, 92, Littré).
[9] For example, *De morbis,* IV, xxxiv (VII, 544 f., Littré), regards the nutrition and growth of plants as a simple process of selecting, by the attraction of like for like, saps existing separately in the soil. The principle of individuation is that of mixture and selection. The chapter is especially interesting for botany and explains the physicians' preference for simples grown in particular places.
[10] *Praef.,* vi and viii, ed. Marx.

first to differentiate them. This view is misleading or, at any rate, inexact.

The treatise on the old school of medicine does, indeed, reject special doctrines (as those of Empedocles), but it insists that medicine is an art or science of long standing and possessed of a recognized and fruitful method by which it has achieved great results and may be expected in the future to advance still farther.[11] Another treatise assures us that medicine is already complete, since it knows the remedies and the proper amounts and times in which to administer them.[12] Medicine, so conceived, was indeed a science and, though limited to a special field, was the peer of the natural philosophy of the day. It might proudly assert that, far from requiring the hypotheses of the natural philosophy, it was only from medicine that one might learn anything about nature.[13]

The truth is, as has already been said, that, except for emphasis and limitations, natural science and medicine were, and remained, essentially one to the time of Aristotle. Aristotle himself says:

> The investigation, too, of the ultimate principles of health and disease is the province of the naturalist: for neither health nor disease can apply to creatures deprived of life. And so it happens, as I think, that most natural philosophers and those physicians who have a more philosophical understanding of their science, end in the one case by investigating medicine and in the other begin with deductions from the laws of nature and their application to medicine.[14]

---

[11] *De prisca medicina*, i (I, 570 f., Littré).
[12] *De locis in homine*, xlvi (VI, 342, Littré).
[13] *De prisca medicina*, i and xx (I, 570 f. and 620 f., Littré).
[14] *De sensu*, 436a, tr. Hammond.

Elsewhere he says:

> It is the province of the physician and also up to a certain point of the natural philosopher to discuss the causes of health and disease, but one must not overlook how they and their subject matter differ. To be sure, what happens bears witness that their fields are up to a point co-terminous; for all the better educated and inquiring physicians discuss the philosophy of nature and derive their principles from it, and the most gifted philosophers almost always in the end lead up to the principles of medicine.[15]

Though the Hippocratics only occasionally refer expressly to philosophers,[16] they are frequently at pains to suggest the philosophical background of their medical views,[17] just as a physician today may by way of introduction allude to fundamental principles of physiology or chemistry which he has no intention of discussing in detail. As Aristotle remarks, the best physicians devote themselves earnestly to knowledge of the body;[18] and it was clearly understood that the human constitution, whatever its composition, was ultimately the same as that of all other things; hence, to know what man is, one must know the nature of the world.[19] Indeed, nothing is more obvious than the assumption which underlies the frequent comparison of the microcosm with the macrocosm and the physical and biological analogies expressly pointed out

---

[15] *De respiratione*, 480b. Cf. *Historia animalium*, 513a.

[16] *De prisca medicina*, xx (I, 620, Littré), to Empedocles; *De natura hominis*, i (VI, 34, Littré), to Melissus.

[17] *De natura mulieris*, i (VII, 312, Littré); *De victu*, I, xxi (VI, 490, Littré); *De carnibus*, i (VIII, 584, Littré); and *De eis quae ad virgines spectant*, i (VIII, 466, Littré).

[18] *Nicomachean Ethics*, 1102a.

[19] See, however, *De prisca medicina*, xx (I, 620, Littré).

or suggested, to wit, that the laws of human physiology are in reality only special forms of universal laws.[20]

This conviction expresses itself also in the view that health and disease depend to a considerable extent on the environment—on climate, water, and locality—and that diseases prove less dangerous if they are akin to general aspects of nature,[21] such as the constitution of the individual, his habit, his age, and the season of the year.[22] Occasionally one is amused by an author's evident desire to show his speculative temper by solemnly declaiming a banal cliché that at the moment was current in philosophical circles, such as "Law governs all things."[23] One could readily match such expressions with similar utterances of physicians today. They are of interest chiefly as demonstrating what every historian already knows, that fundamentally men's minds have changed but little in the course of centuries. The individual differences one readily recognizes among Hippocratics are such as one finds existing among contemporaries in every age, and it is not necessary to assume that they are due to differences in training or background.

To be sure, much is said, for example by Galen, about the Coan and Cnidian schools of medicine and the marks that distinguish one from the other. Certain treatises are usually attributed with assurance to the school of

[20] See note 4 of this chapter. See also *De natura hominis*, vii (VI, 46 f., Littré).
[21] Diocles, frag. 34, Wellmann, disagreed with this view.
[22] *Aphorism.*, II, xxxiv (IV, 480, Littré). The general point of view underlies the excellent treatise *De aere aqua locis*. Cf. Plato, *Timaeus*, 89b f.
[23] *De semine*, i (VII, 490, Littré).

Cnidus,[24] and it is said that they contemplate medicine as a science while the school of Cos, to which Hippocrates belonged, regarded it as an art. Johannes Ilberg, one of the most acute students of the ancient medical literature, says of the putative author of a group of treatises which he pronounces Cnidian:

It is certainly noteworthy that he is not concerned with dogmatically handing down results achieved, but desires to introduce his hearers to the method of scientific investigation. To him explanation is of prime importance, *rerum cognoscere causas*. Here we discover an early stage of serious and genuine investigation. The doctors of Asia Minor and Sicily[25] are among the foremost pioneers in this undertaking.[26]

Without going farther into this question, which is of great importance for the history of Greek medicine, one must admit that the Hippocratic literature is not of a piece, some treatises being frankly concerned only with practice while others reveal a very different temper undoubtedly resembling that of the experimental investigator. The difficulty is that one cannot make a clean separation of the literature into classes corresponding to these "schools."

How this fact is to be accounted for cannot here be considered; it is important, however, not to exaggerate the

[24] For criticism of the Cnidian school by Coan physicians see, for example, *De victu in acutis* (II, 224, Littré); and *Epidem.*, IV, xliii (V, 184, Littré), and VI, iii, 12 (V, 298, Littré).

[25] See Max Wellmann, *Fragmentsammlung der griechischen Aerzte*, Vol. I.

[26] "Die Aerzteschule von Knidos," *Berichte über die Verhandlungen der Sächsischen Akademie der Wissenschaften zu Leipzig, phil.-hist. Klasse*, LXXVI (1924), 12. He refers to the author of *De semine, De natura pueri*, and *De morbis*, IV.

differences and to realize that they do not necessarily imply that the authors belonged to schools fundamentally opposed to one another, because one could readily point to similar disagreement in interest and point of view between modern physicians trained by the same masters. We have always to reckon not only with the school tradition but also, especially in the case of men of outstanding ability, with the natural bent of the individual. This being so, we may for our present purpose disregard the distinction between the schools. Medicine, if it is to meet the daily demands made upon it and improve its practice, must be both an art and a science; but there will always be some who lean more to one of its aspects than to the other and correspondingly contribute more either to theory or to practice.

IV

THE MEDICAL PROFESSION

THE MEDICAL PROFESSION has had a long and honorable career. In the *Odyssey*[1] the doctor was acknowledged to be a "servant of the public" or craftsman on the same footing as others who were treated with respect. The term there employed ($δημιοεργός$) came later indeed to be less honorific, but, if any disparagement was implied in Homeric times, it was only that with which an aristocratic society might regard all who did not belong to it. In the Greece of the sixth and fifth centuries, when social institutions tended more and more toward a purer democracy, the esteem in which physicians were held naturally increased. Meanwhile the art of medicine had advanced, and its practitioners had gained confidence and pride in their profession. In all probability, the position of doctors was similar to that of the seer and the priest. At first they were attached to the households of princes; as the priest was originally the intendant of his private cult, so the doctor was the body-physician of the prince, though he

---

[1] Book XVII, tr. Butcher and Lang: "Whoever himself seeks out and bids to a feast a stranger from afar, save only one of those that are craftsmen of the people, a prophet or a healer of ills, or a shipwright, or even a godlike minstrel, who can delight all with his song."

THE MEDICAL PROFESSION 27

might naturally serve others also, provided that his master required or permitted him to do so. In the transition from royal to democratic rule, characterized by the sway of the Tyrants, one sees, as in the case of Democedes, the court physician emerging as a doctor charged with the care of the public health. Of course, he was not the only one who advised the sick or lent assistance to them, although Greek lands had progressed beyond the stage described by Herodotus as existing in the Orient, where the sick were carried out along the highways and advised by every passer-by. We know that there was in Greece a growing movement among persons of like interests to form associations, clubs, and guilds. We may assume that such existed among physicians; and since the guilds had their "patron saints," the devotees of Apollo and Asclepius (the gods of healing) also would have some such organization. The model of these groups was undoubtedly the ancient clan, with its private cult. Politically, the clans gradually lost their character as closed corporations, but even when they admitted those who were not relations by blood, they were very tenacious of life. Since they traced their lineage back to a god or hero, it may confidently be assumed that they held strongly to an aristocratic tradition. If the court physicians belonged to such guilds they would naturally uphold such a tradition.

In some such way as this we must picture to ourselves the establishment of a code governing the conduct of physicians. Every doctor may be assumed to be familiar with the Hippocratic oath, and one need not, therefore, quote its provisions. It is obvious that it is in the main an aristocratic document, whose motto might properly be *noblesse oblige*. One thinks involuntarily of the oath administered to a squire on becoming a knight. How or when the Hippocratic oath was formulated we have no means of knowing; but there is no reason to suspect that in its essential features it does not represent the ideals of the fifth century B.C. Indeed, it is hard to conceive of it as originating at a later time, when increasing demoralization in public and private life must have made it seem quixotic. It reads as an oath taken by those who are beginning their course of instruction. This fact may contain a suggestion as to its date. It was obviously formulated by physicians. Probability, as well as the statement of Galen, suggests that in the older time the practice of medicine was generally, if not always, transmitted from father to son; by the time of Plato, as the oath also implies, others might be admitted to apprenticeship on payment of fees (and subscribing to articles), a practice which would naturally follow the gradual relaxation of the restriction of membership in the clans, clearly apparent in the sixth and fifth centuries. One seems to sense in the provisions of the oath something more personal than a concern for the integrity of a profession—the determination to guard the honor of the family.

So far as we can see, instruction was personal and individual—there is no evidence of "classes." In the family it would begin at an early age, and the apprentice would naturally attend the doctor in the performance of his duties, just as Cicero learned law by assisting at the consultation of clients with the great jurisconsult, Scaevola. Galen explained the fact that the earliest treatise on anatomy known to him was that of Diocles, a younger contemporary of Aristotle, by saying that textbooks were unnecessary when the apprentice had from youth observed the operations performed by his master. Littré insists that the book alone guarantees the continuity of transmission. More important still, it would seem, is the fact that, while such individual and prolonged instruction may assure the preservation of a definite practice, books, by recording the practice and experiments of different masters, tend to increase of knowledge and by recording different forms of treatment suggest the possibility of still other and better methods.

One of the Hippocratic treatises enlarges on the inconveniences of the doctor's calling, contrasting them with the benefits it confers on his patients.[2] There is a hint of the doctor's sympathy with their sufferings, and it is said that his most difficult task is that of discovering the cause of the complaint. Once that is ascertained, he knows how to proceed. For the most part, however, the doctor utters no complaints on his own account. If detractors of his profession declare that it does not deserve to be called an art or science, he refutes them by pointing out that it has a long and honorable tradition, having an assured method and results to which it can point with pride.[3] To be sure, there are limits set to what the doctor can do; for not all ills can be cured. The doctor cannot be blamed if he foresees the fatal outcome.[4] When he knows that he

[2] *De flatibus*, i (VI, 90, Littré).
[3] *De prisca medicina*, i–iv (I, 570 ff., Littré).
[4] *Prognostic*, i (II, 110 f., Littré).

cannot succeed, he deliberately abstains from the attempt.[5] Disagreement among doctors leads men to doubt the existence of a real art of medicine: some think they are like diviners.[6] Bad doctors, who are doctors only in name, are like supernumerary actors;[7] in fact, most doctors are said to be like bad pilots, good enough in fair weather but likely to cause shipwreck in a storm.[8] Every doctor is of course fallible, but he is to be praised who makes few mistakes. Charlatans, however, are held up to scorn.[9]

Plato was not alone in declaring that there is little certainty, much that is tentative, in medicine, because it is not an exact science defining everything by number and measure;[10] Hippocratic writers repeatedly emphasize this fact.[11] This fact is chiefly due to the doctor's inability to reach the seat of the disease directly and the necessity to infer its nature and cause from symptoms. In certain cases, it is possible by various means to force nature to reveal its secrets;[12] but, especially in its early stages, a disease is often not clearly defined.[13] The treatment also must be in good part tentative or experimental, because

[5] *De morbis*, I, i (VI, 140, Littré); *De arte*, viii (VI, 12, Littré); and Aristotle, *Topica*, 101b.
[6] *De victu in acutis*, iii (II, 240 f., Littré).
[7] *Lex*, i (IV, 638, Littré).
[8] *De prisca medicina*, ix (I, 590, Littré).
[9] *De articulis*, xlii and xliv (IV, 184 and 188, Littré).
[10] *Philebus*, 56a–b. Consequently, much depends upon the experience of the doctor who thereby acquires a semi-instinctive feeling for the course to pursue. Cf. Werner Jaeger, *Diokles von Karystos* (1938), pp. 39 ff.
[11] For example, *De prisca medicina*, ix (I, 588 f., Littré).
[12] *De arte*, x–xii (VI, 16–26, Littré).
[13] *Prognostic*, xx (II, 170, Littré).

THE MEDICAL PROFESSION

there is no objective means of determining the quantity of the remedy to administer. Thus, in giving food, the only test is the feeling of the patients.

It is significant that the Hippocratics should complain of the absence of an objective and absolute standard of amount—either measure, number, or weight.[14] In many cases also the sense of touch furnished the only test, as nurses today may test with the elbow the temperature of the water for a bath. It is clear that the Hippocratics keenly felt the need of a thermometer.[15] But in the dearth or absence of objective tests, since the doctor must know not only what but how much to give, experience must supply the knowledge. Plato insists that to be a physician one must know far more than the medicaments to prescribe.[16] We learn that early doctors used hellebore in too large doses in trying to move the bowels and so caused the death of their patients. This emphasized the need of knowing medicine by practice as well as in theory.[17]

This point of view obviously lays stress on medicine as an art rather than a science. The term τέχνη commonly applied to it would be appropriate to either view, and there were, in fact, some who considered or endeavored to make it a true science, though the Hippocratics clearly thought of it chiefly as an art involving skill and practice as well as knowledge. The emphasis is naturally upon

[14] *De prisca medicina,* ix (I, 588 f., Littré); *De liquidorum usu,* i (VI, 120, Littré); and *De victu,* I, ii (VI, 470, Littré). Plato, *Euthyphro,* 7b–c, emphasizes the thought that one obviates dispute and uncertainty when one can appeal to a definite standard, such as measure, number, or weight.
[15] *De natura hominis,* vii (VI, 46, Littré).
[16] *Phaedrus,* 268a f.
[17] *De articulis,* x (IV, 102, Littré).

knowledge gained by practice and experiment. We have seen that in the time of Hippocrates medical treatises were not rare. The Hippocratic literature is sufficient evidence of this, for in the extant works, numerous as they are, there are references to still others no longer to be found. Hence, we may be sure that such treatises were not neglected. Indeed, we are told that judging the merits of medical literature is an important function of the physician.[18]

How widely these writings were known we have no means of discovering; for some of the works contained in the corpus are plainly notebooks kept by a doctor for his own use, while others are just as clearly compilations from other treatises, hardly more than scrapbooks of excerpts made for future reference. Aristotle knew that the doctor does not learn medicine from books, and he speaks in a way that must precisely express the Hippocratic view. At the close of the *Nicomachean Ethics* he says:

Laws may be set down as the product of the art of politics: how then could one become a legislator from the study of them or judge which of them are the best? For, it appears, men do not become physicians either by the study of books, though their authors undertake to tell not only the remedies but also how one must cure and tend the individuals according to their several conditions. It is commonly believed that such instructions are serviceable to doctors who are experienced, but useless to such as are not. Perhaps, then, collections of laws and constitutions might be useful to those who are able to take a theoretical view and to judge what proposals are good or the reverse, and what measures would fit in with others; but those

---

[18] *Epidem.* III, xvi (III, 100, Littré); *De diebus criticis,* i (IX, 298, Littré).

THE MEDICAL PROFESSION 33

who perused them without that ability could not judge them properly, except by chance, though they might become more capable of understanding (ordinances, once they were proposed).[19]

The comparison between medical treatises and written legislation or constitutions recurs in Aristotle's *Politics*. A question apparently much debated in discussions of the ideal state was whether it were better to be ruled by the best men or by laws. Aristotle decided that it is stupid to determine a course of action by a written code in any art, as the Egyptian law forbade the physician, except at his own peril, to change his mode of treatment within four days.[20] But, he admits, there is another point of view, from which a written constitution may be defended.

We are told that a patient should call in a physician: he will not get better if he is doctored out of a book. But the parallel of the arts is clearly not in point; for the physician does nothing contrary to reason from motives of friendship: he only cures a patient and takes a fee, whereas magistrates do many things from spite and partiality. And, indeed, if a man suspects the physician of being in league with his enemies to destroy him for a bribe, he would rather have recourse to a book. Even physicians, when they are sick, call in other physicians, and training-masters, when they are training, other training-masters, as if they could not judge truly about their own case and might be influenced by their feelings.[21]

One might be tempted to think this attitude the expression of post-Hippocratic times were it not for a passage in Plato where the respective merits of rule by a

[19] 1181a.
[20] *Politica*, 1286a.
[21] *Ibid.*, 1287a, tr. Jowett.

true statesman and under a written code are discussed.[22] If a doctor or a physical trainer, expecting to be absent for a long time, left written directions for those in his charge and then returned unexpectedly, would he, despite changed conditions due to weather or other influences, insist on adhering to his prescription on the ground that that was the only medical and wholesome treatment and every departure from it harmful and contrary to the principles of his art? To do so, we are told, would make medicine or any other art a laughingstock. It is plain both that Aristotle had this discussion in mind and that Plato reflected the established practice of reputable doctors of his time.

These passages make it abundantly clear that recourse to medical treatises was a common practice and show that they contained more than collections of case histories; the treatises distinguished classes of cases and prescribed treatment appropriate to each. One understands, therefore, what the Hippocratics meant by saying that it was an important function of the doctor to judge medical literature, which involves deciding to which class a particular case was to be referred and whether he could approve the treatment recommended for it. Surely, despite the extraordinary advances in the art in the intervening centuries, the problem of the doctor has not essentially changed. These references to medicine on the part of Plato and Aristotle likewise show that it was a representative, if not the representative, art to which one appealed by way of example in trying to decide the rational course of procedure in given circumstances. Plato also says that

[22] *Politicus*, 295.

THE MEDICAL PROFESSION

the physician can give an intelligent reason for everything that he does[23] and that he does everything solely for the good of the whole.[24]

It is plain that Plato had a very high opinion of some doctors, as one infers from many passages besides those already cited. He tells us that because the doctors knows what is good or bad for the well-being of the body medicine must govern, and he contrasts the art of the doctor with arts, such as that of the pastry cook, that pander to men's appetites.[25] Plato speaks of doctors and their assistants, some of whom are slaves and devote themselves to treating slaves, and distinguishes sharply between them. A true physician inquires about the disease from the beginning in the natural way, learning from the patient, imparting his knowledge to the patient and his friends, and instructing the patient to the best of his ability and winning him over to willing coöperation.[26] That this is not an idealized picture is proved by the boast of the rhetorician Gorgias, who claims that he has often gone with his brother, the physician Herodicus, and has by his art persuaded the patient to submit to the required treatment.[27]

All this prepares one to appreciate and accept, as drawn from life, the picture of a true doctor given by Plato.

If one of the slavish empirical doctors were to find a freeman doctor treating a freeman who was sick, talking to him and using arguments closely akin to philosophy, tackling the disease from its origin and showing an understanding of the whole nature of the human body, he would suddenly laugh out loud

---

[23] *Gorgias*, 465a. [24] *Laws*, 902c ff. [25] *Gorgias*, 517e ff.
[26] *Laws*, 720a ff. and 857c. [27] *Gorgias*, 450a–b.

and fall into the language most so-called doctors have at their tongue's ends in such a case, saying, You fool, you are not curing your patient, but instructing him as if he was to become a physician instead of a healthy man.[28]

Let us grant that such doctors were the exception; one might even say, as Plato said of the ideal king, that it would suffice if sometime somewhere such a doctor appeared. One's ideals, as we all know, however high, are only sublimated flesh and blood.

The composite picture of the physician and his art thus obtained may be decorated with a few details. We have a treatise on the doctor's office, giving directions about the apparatus he requires and its arrangement, but we need not go into these details. We know that in many instances he had to treat his patients in their homes or in temporary quarters, for he was likely to wander from place to place. It was not an uncommon occurrence to have another doctor look in and give his opinion of the case or even to engage in a dispute about it with the one in charge, perhaps with a view to supplanting him.[29] Besides, it was not improper to call in other physicians for consultation,[30] just as the doctor, when sick, called in a colleague to assume control, in order to make sure of an objective view of the case.

In the heterogeneous mass of Hippocratic literature there are occasional hints of regard for the opinion of the ignorant vulgar;[31] but on the whole the tone is severely professional.

[28] *Laws,* 857c.
[29] *De morbis,* I, i (VI, 140 f., Littré).
[30] *Praecepta,* vii–viii (IX, 261–65, Littré).
[31] *De articulis,* lxvii, 70 (IV, 288, Littré).

THE MEDICAL PROFESSION 37

It is disgraceful in every art, especially in medicine, to make much ado, create a great spectacle, and indulge in much talk, and then accomplish no good result.[32]

The most important thing in every branch of the art is to make well what is diseased; if it can be done in more ways than one, one must choose the simplest, for that is both most humane and most in accordance with the art, unless, of course, one hankers for specious mystification.[33]

The rule is: be helpful to the patient; at any rate, do him no harm.[34] An important injunction is to guard against injurious aftereffects of the treatment.[35]

The intellectual outlook of the Hippocratics is clear enough; they were obviously the peers of the best minds in the Greece of their time, as is shown among other things by the community of interest they had with the philosophers. However much individuals might object to the intrusion of too rash speculations of certain philosophers in the medical art,[36] the spirit in which they approached their problems and their cases was thoroughly scientific. If they failed to appreciate the complexity of the matters they had to deal with and at times imagined that they had all but attained perfection, one who recalls the extravagant dreams of certain eminent scientists in our day will be loath to blame them. Success even in small things causes elation that only a cynic will despise. The aim of the Hippocratics was to make medicine thoroughly scientific. Perhaps not all would have shared the enthu-

[32] *Ibid.*, xliv (IV, 188, Littré).
[33] *Ibid.*, lxxviii (IV, 312, Littré).
[34] *Epidem.*, I, v (II, 634, Littré).
[35] *De affectionibus*, xiii (VI, 220, Littré).
[36] See *De natura hominis*, i (VI, 32, Littré).

siastic declaration of one writer that the philosophic doctor was the peer of the gods or his contention that one must carry philosophy into medicine and medicine into philosophy;[37] but few, one fancies, would object to the exhortation of another: "Endeavor to be a scientist, observing closely the condition and strength of your patient."[38] In keeping with such ideals are the intellectual capacities demanded of the would-be physician.

Finally, moral requisites of a high standard were recommended, if not exacted, by the Hippocratics. It is hardly necessary to recall the virtues mentioned in the Hippocratic oath and in the *Physician*: it suffices to say that they do not differ from those demanded of a doctor today.[39] Human nature being what it is, one is certain that there were lapses in ancient times as there are today. One Hippocratic actually relates how he deliberately brought about what he mistakenly thought to be an abortion,[40] a practice forbidden by the oath. A modern doctor would not publicly declare that he had done so, though we know that despite strict legal prohibition the practice has not ceased. We think of ourselves as having a Christian civilization, though the Christian virtues are perhaps more honored in the breach than in the observance. The im-

---

[37] *De decenti habitu*, iv (IX, 232, Littré).

[38] *De sterilibus mulieribus*, ccxxx (VIII, 442, Littré).

[39] An interesting point is the professional, rather than a mercenary, attitude in the matter of doctor's fees—the doctor's "philanthropic" motives. See *Praecepta*, vi (IX, 258, Littré). Galen, *De placitis Hippocratis et Platonis*, V, 751, Kühn, rebuking Menedotus for saying that the practice of medicine was a business like any other, declared that all the great physicians, among them Hippocrates and Diocles, were moved by love of man, not by love of fame or gain.

[40] *De natura pueri*, xiii (VII, 490, Littré).

portant thing, meanwhile, is that an ideal be held before us, however feebly we may exert ourselves to realize it in our conduct. Well might a historian of medicine say:

Had the Hippocratic writings done nothing during more than two thousand years but waken and keep alive in countless individuals the sense of the dignity of the medical art and the honor of the profession, they would deserve on that account alone to be blessed by the latest generations.[41]

If one were asked to single out the most profound observation in the Hippocratic literature, one might well be at a loss. One reader has, however, found much food for thought in the casual remark that there are three factors concerned in every case: the disease, the patient, and the doctor.[42] The more one reflects upon it, the more significant it becomes. The physician is the servant of his art; the patient must fight the disease with the help of the doctor. Always, but especially in desperate cases, the help the doctor renders is largely spiritual; only a true man can give it.

[41] Haeser, *Lehrbuch der Geschichte der Medicin*, I, 210.
[42] *Epidem.*, I, i, 5 (II, 636, Littré). Cf. *Aphorism.*, I, i (IV, 458, Littré).

V

SOME SCIENTISTS OF THE DAY

THUS FAR we have been chiefly concerned with the general outlook of the Hippocratics. It is clear that they shared the intellectual interests of their time, and, unless all signs deceive us, physicians were among the foremost representatives of the scientific and philosophic movements from the sixth century onwards. If one has not always recognized their part in these movements, the failure to do so can with probability be explained by a number of circumstances that call for remark. It has already been pointed out that in the earlier stages of Greek science its devotees were not sharply differentiated. One either was, or was not, a man of science. To be sure there had been "healers" (ἰατροί) from Homeric times; but though there were individuals of recognized and special skill, the profession as a closed corporation was of considerably later date. The name also, like that of the "sage" (σοφός), the "philosopher," and the "naturalist," still awaited definition. One sees in Plato's *Apology of Socrates*[1] how even Socrates, the ironical sage of Foxtown, sought, somewhat as one turns to a dictionary, for the

[1] 21b ff.

meaning of the Delphic oracle which had declared there was no man wiser than he. Terms and functions were still fluid. As Aristotle remarked, physicians in the end touched on philosophy, and philosophers, if they were clever and followed out their principles, had in the end to concern themselves with medicine.[2]

In the strictly scientific aspects of his thinking, Aristotle was obviously deeply indebted to the medical tradition—how much we can never fully know—while for his "first philosophy" and the interests that grew out of and grouped themselves about it he was to all intents and purposes essentially a Platonist. To the time of Plato science had been one. Plato's interest, to be sure, as was natural to a devoted follower of Socrates, was directed principally to ethical, logical, and metaphysical problems, but he made no hard and fast distinctions. In the group of works centering in the *Republic* he obviously intended to redress the balance, for it is clear that the *Critias* was conceived as an essay in the field of history and geography and the *Timaeus* as one covering the ground of the traditional treatises *On Nature*. *Timaeus* was completed but was apparently not taken very seriously by its author, however highly it was esteemed by later Platonists; *Critias* was left unfinished one may be sure for the simple reason that it could not hold his interest.

Aristotle stood at the parting of the ways; he was by nature and in intention a Summist, but he made a beginning in distinguishing fields and treating of them in separate works. In his school, as we have seen, was made the first thoroughgoing attempt at a separation, when Theo-

[2] See p. 22.

phrastus undertook to sketch the history of natural philosophy, Menon the history of medicine, and Eudemus that of mathematics, astronomy, and theology.

From this delimitation of fields some curious and instructive results followed, partly because of the attempted definition of terms, partly because Aristotle himself had somehow classified the thinkers. Thus, to cite an example, Aristotle had thought (and perhaps called[3]) the Eleatics "unnatural" philosophers but had cited Parmenides and Melissus in regard to matters that are concerned with the physical world, whereas he mentioned nothing of the sort in connection with Zeno. Accordingly, Parmenides and Melissus, but not Zeno, figure in the doxographic tradition that goes back ultimately to Theophrastus. Whatever else one may infer from the omission of Zeno, it is plain that we have here an undoubted result of the Aristotelian influence.

A similar case, in another category, is that of Alcmaeon. Though he apparently was chiefly interested in physiology[4] and was certainly a physician, he had touched upon other problems that occupied the attention of the natural philosophers, and Aristotle had taken note of his opinions. Hence he figures prominently in the doxographic tradition and passes currently as a philosopher. Theophrastus himself dutifully included him in his account, though one cannot determine how much of that given by Aëtius is actually derived from his historical sketch. Since comparatively little concerning him comes to us directly through the medical line of tradition, this rather para-

---
[3] Sextus Empiricus, *Adv. Mathem.*, X, xlvi.
[4] Diels, V, i. 210, 15.

SOME SCIENTISTS OF THE DAY 43

doxical situation makes Alcmaeon a difficult person to place.

The difficulty is increased by uncertainty as to his date and connections. We know that he lived at Croton in southern Italy, where there was a strong Pythagorean society; and he has been claimed as a Pythagorean, though without good reason. Aristotle did not know whether he influenced Pythagoreans or was influenced by them, and the grounds for suggesting either possibility are so trivial that they count for nothing. Alcmaeon is generally dated early in the fifth century because of a statement included in inferior manuscripts of Aristotle but omitted by the best manuscript and apparently unknown to Alexander Polyhistor. In all probability the statement in question is a later addition to the text of Aristotle taken from Porphyry's *Life of Pythagoras*. We are, therefore, without dependable evidence regarding either his date or his connections. Judging by his opinions, one would naturally take him for an unusually intelligent physician living about 450 B.C. and without recognizable affiliation with any special group of natural philosophers.[5] He seems rather to have been the typical man of science of the time,

[5] I have discussed the record in the *American Journal of Philology*, LXI (January, 1940), 3 ff. It is true that Alcmaeon addressed his book to three fellow townsmen of Croton, who were reported to have been Pythagoreans; but this connection actually proves nothing more than a personal relation. As regards the date of Alcmaeon, we have no satisfactory evidence. To be sure, one of the three men to whom he addressed his book, Bro[n]tinus, figures in the Pythagoras legend as the husband or father of Theano, who is variously reported to have been the pupil or wife of Pythagoras. Spurious letters were attributed to her. Clearly, nothing can be inferred from such data. Scholars are agreed that the Pythagorean scheme of ten pairs of contraries, with which Aristotle compared the contraries of Alcmaeon without deciding which preceded

interested in all aspects of scientific investigation and speculation but chiefly devoted to physiology.

It will, therefore, repay one to give attention to this man as an example of the ideals and methods of the medical profession in the generation just preceding that of Hippocrates. Like certain Hippocratics he sought to display his interest in the current problems of general science by (apparently) occasional remarks about cosmological matters. Thus he is reported to have held that the moon and all that lies beyond it are eternal.[6] As to the planets, we are told that he agreed with certain "mathematicians" in asserting that they have a motion contrary to that of the fixed stars, moving from west to east.[7] The sun is flat, and the phases and obscuration of the moon he explained, like Heraclitus and Antiphon, by the turning of its skifflike body[8] Aristotle says that Alcmaeon held views regarding the soul similar to those of Thales, Diogenes of Apollonia, and Heraclitus, asserting that the soul is immortal because it resembles things immortal, as being continually in motion, for all things divine are continually in motion—sun, stars, and the whole heaven.[9] In this sense we are doubtless to understand the statement of the pseudo-Aristotelian *Problems* that Alcmaeon said men perish because they cannot (like the stars that move in circles) join the end to the beginning.[10] This is highly speculative, as is much that we find in other early thinkers. There are not wanting significant obser-

---

the other, was of late origin, dating presumably after 450 B.C. The books attributed to Bro[n]tinus, also, were either spurious or of questionable origin.

[6] Diels, V, i, 210, 18.   [7] *Ibid.*, 19 ff.
[8] *Ibid.*, 32.   [9] *Ibid.*, 213, 17 ff. Cf. *Ibid.*, 210, 21.   [10] *Ibid.*, 215, 4 f.

vations, such as that regarding the apparently retrograde motion of the planets, but they do not serve to date Alcmaeon. The "mathematicians" who are said to have held the same views were presumably Pythagoreans, but of what date we do not know.[11] It has been claimed that Alcmaeon's belief that the soul is immortal was due to Pythagorean influence. It is true that Aristotle elsewhere cites Pythagoreans as holding that the soul is continually in motion,[12] and we know that they believed in its immortality. But these doctrines were not peculiar to them, and it is noteworthy that Aristotle did not assert Alcmaeon's agreement with them but rather with Thales, Diogenes of Apollonia, and Heraclitus.[13] When he reported that some Pythagoreans identified the soul with the motes in the sunbeam he had in mind a comparison of Pythagoreans with the Atomists.[14] It is important to emphasize these points because unwarranted conclusions have been drawn from inconclusive data. There is in fact nothing specifically Pythagorean in what we know of his opinions. Once we recognize this fact we are prepared to see him in his true role, as a man of intelligence interested in all the problems of his time and therefore as a representative of the period to which he belonged.

As we have noted, Alcmaeon is said to have written chiefly on medical matters, though he occasionally touched

---

[11] The comparison of views here suggested is probably due to the rearrangement of the data furnished by Theophrastus, whose account dealt with thinkers seriatim. When the views of the thinkers were broken into fragments and distributed according to subject matter, as they were by Aëtius, there resulted comparisons and contrasts from which we cannot draw any conclusions regarding a possible historical connection.
[12] Diels, V, i, 462, 26.
[13] Ibid., 213, 17 f.
[14] Ibid., 462, 29 ff.

on questions of a general scientific or philosophical character. He owes his importance chiefly to his medical and physiological studies. The emphasis on pairs of opposite states or qualities, which led Aristotle to bring him into comparison with certain Pythagoreans who set up a table of ten pairs of opposites,[15] we may be sure was part of his medical doctrine. There is in fact no point of contact between the two groups of opposites mentioned in our sources except "the good and the bad," which obviously is too much a commonplace to be significant, and one naturally concludes that Aristotle suggested a possible relation between them only because Alcmaeon resided at Croton where the Pythagorean order had its principal seat. The notion of regarding things as arranged in contrasting groups is so natural, especially to the Greeks,[16] that it is idle to speculate who may have originated it. In medicine, in particular, it was doubtless a primitive practice to combat a diseased condition by inducing its opposite—to fight heat with cold and cold with heat.[17] Heraclitus had seen all nature as such a battle, and in Greek medicine a physician was always thought of as fighting a peccant substance or condition. The most that one may infer, therefore, is that Alcmaeon was the first or most prominent medical writer known to Aristotle who emphasized this opinion.

It is certain that Alcmaeon based his medical practice on this notion; for we know that he regarded health as due to the equilibrium ($\iota\sigma o\nu o\mu\iota a$) of the elements compos-

---

[15] *Ibid.*, 211, 11 ff.
[16] See Burnet, *Early Greek Philosophy*, p. 8.
[17] Aristotle, *Nicomachean Ethics*, 1104b, and Plato, *Phaedo*, 86b f.

SOME SCIENTISTS OF THE DAY 47

ing the body, whereas the sway of one among them (μοναρχία) produces disease.[18] The terms ἰσονομία and μοναρχία, if actually used by Alcmaeon, mark the application of politico-social concepts to the physical sphere, as had already been done by Anaximander and Heraclitus and was continued, among others, by Empedocles, who was presumably his contemporary.[19]

How Alcmaeon thought of the constituents of the body we are unable to gather from our sources, but we may probably assume that they were for him definite substances possessing characteristic properties. The terms in which their relations to one another are expressed suggest a conflict not unlike that presupposed by Anaximander and proclaimed by Heraclitus and Empedocles. In the history of medical thought few notions are so persistent as that of a war within our members, and it has its analogy in religion and ethics as the conflict between good and evil. There is no dating such conceptions; certainly neither Alcmaeon nor the Pythagoreans originated the notion that the physician comes to the aid of the patient in his struggle against the evil forces of disease.

Thus far there is nothing to mark Alcmaeon as exceptional. He was, nevertheless, a pioneer of outstanding merit; for, so far as we know, he was the first to undertake dissection of animals in the service of physiology. Chalcidius presumably thought he actually practiced vivisection,[20] but we need not accept his view. Alcmaeon's

[18] Diels, V, i, 215, 11 ff.
[19] Anaximander regarded the excess of one factor or phase of the cosmic order or process as injustice, and the notion of an overruling decree of justice (δίκη) is prominent in his thought, as in that of Empedocles. [20] Diels, V, i, 212, 23.

principal interest appears to have been directed to discovering the seat of intelligence and the channels of communication to it from the sense organs. Theophrastus says that he distinguished between sense perception and intelligence, claiming that the other animals perceive with the senses but man alone understands.[21] He appears to have inferred that the brain must be the seat of intelligence from the observation that if it suffers concussion all the senses (and, of course, the intellect also) are impaired. The senses must, therefore, be connected with the brain; and he dissected animals to discover and trace the connection. This he found in certain "pores," or channels, which he traced from eyes and ears to the brain. When perception is interrupted or impaired, he thought, it is because these channels are obstructed. He offered explanations, based on his findings, of sight and hearing which long continued to influence thought on these subjects. His explanations of taste and smell were vague, presumably because he did not discover the "channels" from their organs to the brain. The nerves he sought were not so easily traced. The same is, of course, the case with the general sensory nerves; and we are told by Theophrastus that he offered no explanation of the sense of touch.[22]

Aside from his investigation of the sense organs and the brain, we receive information chiefly of his views regarding sexual reproduction and embryology. These need not detain us here, since they were in general like those of his contemporaries; but it is to be noted that he was obviously in these matters, as in regard to the senses,

[21] *Ibid.*, 211, 35 ff.
[22] *Ibid.*, 212, 9. Cf. Theophrastus, *De sensu* (Diels, *Doxographi Graeci*, pp. 500 ff.), on Plato.

basing his conclusions on personal observation and dissection. Alcmaeon, we discover, was an experimentalist; and in this also, though he may have been outstanding, he did not stand alone.

His (perhaps younger) contemporaries Empedocles and Anaxagoras followed the same method. Empedocles was a physician, he is even regarded as the founder of the Sicilian school of medicine. It is doubtful whether one may properly speak of a Sicilian school, though Empedocles unquestionably exercised a considerable influence on physicians of the latter half of the fifth century, chiefly because he more definitely formulated the conception of physical elements, or "roots," as he called them. In a strict sense, indeed, these "roots" were not elements as we understand the term, but rather (to use the language of Lucretius) *maxima mundi membra,* the principal masses of matter composing the world. Empedocles, like others who adopted his classification of matter, was well aware that earth, for example, was not uniform but differed widely in character and composition; and though at the nodal points of the cosmic process he imagined the four "roots" as momentarily separated, he believed that in the world as we know it they were intimately combined in different proportions.

As regards the actual state of the world, there was little to choose between the mixture of "roots" in his theory and the "all things together" of his contemporary Anaxagoras. Anaxagoras, whether or not a practicing physician, was obviously preoccupied with physiological problems: indeed, his theory was due chiefly to his attempt to explain the phenomena of the nutrition and growth of organic beings. We have no reason to go at length into the philosophies of these two important thinkers; but it is important to note that both experimented with a view to explaining physiological processes.

To Empedocles we owe an explanation of the process of respiration illustrated by the action of the water clock,[23] and we know that Anaxagoras also occupied himself with the same instrument, doubtless because of his interest in the same problem. Anaxagoras experimented also with inflated bags, proving that air is not the absence of matter but a corporeal substance. The water clock, moreover, offered an explanation of other physiological phenomena, such as the circulation of the blood that conditions nutrition of all the parts of the body. The body being porous, and therefore capable of admitting substances in suitable form, the question arose how the necessary movement was brought about. The experiment with the water clock showed that when air escaped water flowed in to replace it and vice versa. This was the process afterwards called by Erasistratus "pursuit of the evacuated," or *horror vacui*.

The Hippocratics explained the circulation from organ to organ on the same principle, partly on the analogy of the cupping glass, partly on that of vessels with communicating tubes. How the process was conceived as starting is not expressly stated, though we may reasonably infer that it was supposed to be due to the native heat of the body. Anaxagoras explained the creation of the organs by the native heat of the fetus,[24] no doubt assum-

[23] Frag. 100, Diels.
[24] Diels, V, ii, 30, 33 f.

ing that it expanded the inclosed air and thus forced passages that developed into veins, etc. That heat causes a flow of air was known and illustrated by the flickering of a flame (as of a candle) in a closed room.[25] The Hippocratics frequently employ the conception of the attraction of humors by heat caused by inflammation. All these processes were familiar to them and they were obviously connected in the thought of the medical writers of the fifth century and were illustrated by phenomena observable in familiar things. If we may accept as true the anecdote told by Plutarch about the goat with a single horn,[26] which the soothsayer regarded as a portent, Anaxagoras must also have practiced dissection; for he is reported to have examined the skull of the animal and discovered the cause of the anomalous phenomenon in the abnormal deflection of the growth.

Still another philosopher of the latter half of the fifth century calls for mention. Diogenes of Apollonia exercised an influence on the Hippocratics second to none. How great that influence was, and in what particulars it is to be detected, is, however, in part debatable; for Diogenes was only one of a large number of men of his time who were speculating and investigating along similar lines. To what chance he owed the prominence he enjoys in the record, while others, perhaps more original, have remained unnoticed, we cannot say. One can only guess that the attention paid to him by the comic poets may have had something to do with it. Whether he was a practicing physician is uncertain; but he was, like most

---

[25] *De carnibus*, vi (VIII, 592, Littré).
[26] *Pericles*, vi; Diels, V, ii, 10, 26 f.

thinkers of his time, much concerned with physiological problems. Aristotle mentioned his views a few times, and Theophrastus dealt at length with his physiology of the senses. This insured his inclusion in the doxographic tradition and his standing as a "philosopher." Simplicius, to whom we owe most of the authentic fragments of Diogenes' writings, so regarded him, but what he reports throws little light on his connections; for he says that he borrowed some doctrines from Anaxagoras and others from Leucippus.[27] We cannot point out any influence of Leucippus; if there was any, we may suspect that it was in his cosmology. His dependence on Anaxagoras, however, is plain, and quite as evident is the debt he owed to Anaximenes of the old school of Miletus in the emphasis he laid on the role of air both in cosmology and physiology.

One treatise in the Hippocratic corpus, *De flatibus*, must be chiefly a restatement of the views of Diogenes. According to its author, air is the controlling agent in the body, as in the world at large. Other physicians shared essentially the same views, though they spoke of πνεῦμα, *spiritus*, rather than of air. The earlier adherents of the pneuma doctrine appear to have made no distinction between pneuma and the air we breathe; but later, especially by Aristotle and those under his influence, the pneuma, regarded as a cause of disease, was defined as a περίττωμα, a surplusage or residue of digestion or other physiological process. If Aristotle was wont, as is reported,[28] to go to bed with a flask of hot oil laid over his

---

[27] Diels, V, ii, 52, 30 f.
[28] Diogenes Laërtius, V, xvi. See *De flatibus*, ix (VI, 104, Littré): hot poultices relieve flatulence. See also *Regimen in acutis*, vii (II, 268 f., Littré).

SOME SCIENTISTS OF THE DAY 53

stomach, his emphasis on that aspect of pneuma is understandable. We need not dwell longer on the medical views of Diogenes; but it is important to recall that Aristotle quoted at length his description of the system of veins.[29] Although the superficial veins are chiefly considered, it is evident that he must have dissected animals, by that time a common practice. Systematic anatomy, thus prepared, was notably advanced by Aristotle, Diocles, Erasistratus, and Herophilus.

Toward the close of the fifth century there was apparently a revival of the philosophy of Heraclitus. In several of the Hippocratic treatises, notably in *De victu*, Book I, and *De nutrimento,* the influence of this school, even more that of the enigmatic and antithetical style of Heraclitus himself, is plainly to be seen. It cannot be said that the school contributed much to medical thought, but it served to emphasize a conception that was already latent in the practice and theory of Greek medicine. Plato said that according to the Thracians one cannot cure the body without beginning with the soul, whence all flows, and that good physicians maintained that in order to heal the eyes one must cure the head and, indeed, the whole body.[30] In referring to the Thracians he was thinking of the "charms" they were supposed to use; but the "good doctors" were doubtless Greeks. It is a notable fact that the Hippocratics, in respect to therapy, have comparatively little to say of separate parts or organs of the body;

---

[29] Frag. 6, Diels.
[30] *Charmides,* 156b. Classical writers had much to say of the charms used by the Thracians. Socrates playfully pretends to have been taught their use by a Thracian.

their attention was always directed chiefly to the body as a whole, and they were not unmindful of the mental condition of their patients. It was, therefore, nothing new, though it was important, to stress the conception that the physiological functions form a unity, and that a disease, wherever it may have its principal seat, must affect the entire organism.

It is true that, in general, the Hippocratics rejected the monistic doctrines of certain philosophers,[31] who held that man, like all other bodies, was constituted of a single element, although, as we have seen, *De flatibus* attributed all diseases to the influence of air. They also rejected the notion that a single humor was the cause of all disorders. The doctor must indeed know the components of the body, and the emphasis was generally on the humors. Much as one may condemn the theory of the four humors, which had so long a vogue, one cannot fail to recognize the value of the emphasis upon the fluids of the body. Not only was this natural, because the Greek physicians were chiefly concerned with acute diseases and because the more stable parts of the body are less liable to disease, but the humors, as fluids, were recognized as penetrating the solid structure and therefore affecting the whole.

This fundamental concept is the theme of the treatises *De victu*, Book I, and *De nutrimento*. Using Heraclitean language and imagery, they point out the instability and reciprocal interchange in cosmos and microcosm, in body and mind. One may perhaps paraphrase the general conception in the statement of *De nutrimento:* "All things

[31] See, for example, *De natura hominis*, i (VI, 32 f., Littré).

conspire together as one, all flow together in a single confluence, all suffer in sympathy, each with other."[32] On this view the physician must direct his attention to the whole—not only to the whole body but also to the mind and to the environment. If this is philosophical rather than specifically medical, it is a profound philosophy which the physician must share. It means, among other things, that a patient's condition cannot be safely judged by noting a few isolated symptoms. How circumspect some of the Hippocratics were may be inferred from the following passage:

Sum up what you can ascertain about the origin and onset of the disorder from frequent converse [with your patient and his friends?], and what you discover little by little; put all together, and find out whether all the points agree, and also, if some points do not fit into the picture, whether these agree among themselves, so that a single likeness may result from the differing symptoms. That is the true method. In this way you will confirm what is right and disprove what is wrong in your diagnosis.[33]

The full significance of this statement may not be at once apparent. That it contemplates a unified picture[34] composed of all the data obtainable will be appreciated by every doctor. That demand is at the root of all science and philosophy. How one comes to make that demand in a world seemingly so confused and recalcitrant is a fair question. There are those who regard it as a moral

---

[32] Cap. xxiii (IX, 106, Littré).
[33] *Epidem.*, VI, iii, 12 (V, 298, Littré). Cf. *De officina medici,* i (III, 272, Littré).
[34] *De officina medici,* i (III, 272, Littré); and *Prorrhetic,* II, iii (IX, 10 ff., Littré).

postulate, and, certainly, rational conduct is impossible except on the assumption of an order and a unity underlying the manifold disarray that seems everywhere to confront us. To become intelligible and admit of rational treatment the facts must be somehow reduced to order; but any pattern we may fashion is apt to be incomplete, leaving some data to plague us, and the more one goes into details the more numerous are the parts that refuse to be included in the picture. These, the unintelligible factors in the situation, constitute the real challenge to understanding, and it is only by combining them into an acceptable pattern that one can satisfy the demand for an intelligible order—in a word, for understanding. It is interesting to see this ancient physician so clearly conscious of the intellectual process; if one misses anything in his statement, it is the suggestion that the existence of recalcitrant factors is a challenge to renewed inquiry, to the discovery of further facts that may help to integrate the whole. This omission, indeed, is not accidental; for the principal difference between ancient and modern science is, perhaps, that modern science is more conscious of the need of discovering more facts and employs systematic experimentation to bring them to light. We must remember, however, that we are now dealing not with a worker in a medical institute or laboratory but with a practicing physician at the bedside of a patient. He has to act promptly on such knowledge as is immediately available; he is well aware that the art is long and time is fleeting and that at best what he can do is tentative, because he can see in part only.[35]

[35] *Aphorism.*, i (IV, 458, Littré).

VI

SCIENTIFIC METHODS

IF ONE ATTEMPTS a systematic survey of the Hippocratic literature, one is baffled not only by its mass but also by the varied contents of the several treatises. The arrangement of the works according to subject matter presents not a little difficulty. Perhaps Haeser's arrangement is as good as any. But it soon becomes evident that Hippocratic medicine cannot without violence be subjected to the categories usual in modern medical handbooks. For our present purpose such an arrangement of the matters to be considered would be useless as well as inappropriate, because it must emphasize results, which, though historically interesting, do not adequately measure the significance of the pioneers. In some domains—for example, in surgery—the achievements of the Hippocratics were notable indeed, and certain of their procedures may even now be followed with advantage; but if one approaches them in the hope of learning new facts, one will generally be disappointed. Their knowledge of the human body and of the specific causes of disease was, in comparison with that obtainable today, so meager that the modern reader who appraises their worth by that standard is apt to be appalled by their shortcomings. Thus the physiology of the healthy body was little known, and the attention of the physician was directed chiefly to the departure in disease from the normal as observed on the surface, which was familiar because of the opportunities afforded by gymnastic exercises. Anatomy, except such as could be learned from occasional wounds, was in the Hippocratic age generally limited to inferences drawn from the dissection of lower animals. Hippocratic knowledge of the bones, to be had from skeletons, was on the whole exact; that of the nerves, muscles, and tissues, excepting such as was required for surgery, was either inadequate or wanting—for example, even the distinction between veins and arteries is not quite certain. The important organs were known to them, but their functions were in some cases wholly misconceived, as when the brain was believed to be the source of phlegm. As for the causes of diseases, they were aware of influences exerted by injuries and other external agencies, such as climate, changes of temperature, seasons, waters, and miasmas and also by excesses or deficiencies in nutrition and the manner of life. Naturally, they were ignorant of the specific causes revealed by microbiology; and the absence or deficiency of certain elements supplied by vitamins was, of course, likewise unknown. In their humoral pathology there was, however, explicit recognition of relative deficiency, because the predominance of one humor, which was thought to cause disease, must be at the expense of others.[1]

Obviously, then, the merits of Hippocratic medicine are

[1] See *De flatibus*, i (VI, 92, Littré); *Aphorism.*, II, xxii (IV, 476, Littré); and Diocles, frags. 41, 43, 48, 70, and 77, Wellmann.

SCIENTIFIC METHODS 59

not to be found in the detailed knowledge of the body and the specific causes of its disorders. Such knowledge as the physician had he owed essentially to experience gained in his practice, which taught him to judge the presumable course of a disease and the means best suited to overcome it. His success must depend in good part on the natural curative force of the body,[2] which he supports to the best of his ability while countering the effects of the disorder.[3] Plato represents[4] Eryximachus, a physician, the son of the physician Acumenus, as saying in his praise of love, that there are in the body, as in the mind and in all other things human and divine, two loves—one of the healthy, one of the sickly state; it is honorable and decorous to indulge the former and thwart the latter.

Medicine, in fact, is the science of the body's loves with reference to repletion and evacuation; and he who in these matters can diagnose the beautiful and the ugly love will be the ablest doctor. And hence the man who can effect a transformation, so that instead of the one love the other is acquired; he who understands the method of implanting love in bodies where no love exists and where one must come into being, and how to extirpate a love that is within; this man no doubt would be a good practitioner.[5]

He must be able to reconcile the elements of the body that are most opposed to one another and thus to bring

---

[2] *De prisca medicina,* xvi (I, 606 f., Littré); and *Epidem.,* VI, v, 1 (V, 314, Littré).
[3] Diseases cured by their opposites, *De flatibus,* i (VI, 92, Littré); Aristotle, *Nicomachean Ethics,* 1104b; and [Aristotle], *Problem.,* 866b.
[4] In the *Symposium.*
[5] *Symposium,* 186b f., tr. Lane Cooper.

about a harmony or concord where there was war. Except for the imaginative form, the statement might be accepted as the doctrine of the Hippocratics, of all Greek medical writers from Alcmaeon onwards.

Haeser well says:

The imperishable fame of the Hippocratics rests on the firm foundation of the spirit that pervades their therapy—their reasonable reflection on the object to be achieved, accurate definition of the attainable, calm assurance and care in carrying out the treatment. What has been tested and approved by long experience is always preferred to the spectacular and the new.[6]

This applies to practice; but we need to inquire what lay behind and justified their confidence. Of course it was experience, and such experience is not the result of haphazard observation.

The foundation of all science is observation. That the Greeks, in particular the Greek physicians, were keen observers is too well known to call for special remark. The best evidence is to be found in the casebooks, of which there are many in the Hippocratic literature. There is, however, nothing singular about mere observation, however keen; it is not peculiar to man, and perhaps the more primitive races surpass in this respect the more highly civilized. The recording of observations is a step in advance, because it implies the recognition of their importance. Here, also, the Greeks were not the pioneers, for records of observations had long been kept by Egyptians and Babylonians, though their interest was not al-

[6] Vol. I, p. 159. He refers to *Aphorism.*, II, lii (IV, 484, Littré), and *De fracturis*, i (III, 412 f., Littré).

ways in our sense scientific. A most striking example of Greek observation and record in the field of medicine is the description of the great plague at Athens left by Thucydides,[7] a contemporary of Hippocrates. He states that he himself had been smitten by it and gives his reason for recording the symptoms and course of the disease—that it may be recognized if it should ever recur. A comparable record might be made of a new species of plants or animals, a description enabling one to identify it whenever or wherever its like was found. From the Hippocratic treatises one could cite a number of singularly minute descriptions of a single disease or a concourse of diseases.

One of these concerns an epidemic of coughing at Perinthus,[8] which Littré identified as diphtheria, while others have thought it might have been several diseases combining to assail the region. If a doubt remains as to the identity of the epidemic, it is hardly the fault of the Hippocratic practitioner, but it is probably due to the well-known circumstance that diseases change in the course of time. Valuable as such observations are, they would, of course, need to be supplemented for the doctor by experience, either his own or that of others; for a description of the symptoms, however accurate, need not result in a true diagnosis or suggest the proper cure. Owing to the limitations of their knowledge, the diagnosis of the Hippocratics cannot have compared favorably with that of today.

The fact that in many instances—for example, in the *Epidemics*—no mention of the treatment is included in the

[7] See II, xlviii ff.
[8] *Epidem.*, VI, vii, 1 (V, 330 f., Littré).

casebooks has led some writers on Greek medicine to think of the Hippocratics as heartless bystanders who did nothing but record what they saw. Thucydides also says nothing of the means employed in combating the plague. Why in this instance he was merely a reporter one cannot say with assurance; but it goes without saying that in all cases, as in that of the plague, the doctors tried every means they could think of; for Thucydides records that the mortality was especially great among them because they attended the sick. Surely the prayers and incantations which he mentions as having been finally abandoned were not the only expedients resorted to.[9] The Hippocratics are remarkably free from superstitious practices and decry them.

However important the mere observation and recording of fact may be in the furtherance of pure science, the medical practitioner, who is bound to act without unnecessary delay, must direct his attention to symptoms, that is to say, to significant phenomena. This implies a valuation of things to be observed such as, if true, can be based only on experience. That the Hippocratics commanded a fund of experience sufficient to enable them to distinguish between what was important and what one might neglect is abundantly shown by the repeated instructions regarding the factors of which one must take account in one's reckoning. Every selection is, of course, contingent on one's purpose. The ultimate object of the practitioner was naturally mastery over disease, and, just as inevitably, the proximate purpose was to determine its

---

[9] Cf. Plutarch, *De Iside et Osiride*, 383b, and Acron, frag. 6, Wellmann.

cause.[10] Because of their limited knowledge of physiology and their total ignorance of microbiology, one will not expect to find in the Hippocratics satisfactory answers to the difficult and complicated questions that are still confronting the medicine of our day. Indeed, one discovery, however important, apparently only opens up further questions. What one has a right to demand of a science is that it approach its problems in a rational and clearsighted way.

In this respect, the Hippocratics will not be found wanting; for they recognized the fundamental fact that in dealing with disease one must take account not only of the individual and his constitution, character, and habits[11] but also of more general factors, such as the race and sex of the patient and the environment—climate, location, and water supply and even social and political conditions. However important consideration of the general factors must be in regard to problems of general public health, the Hippocratics, though sometimes confronted with endemic or epidemic conditions, were chiefly concerned with the individual patient. Nothing is more characteristic of Hippocratic medicine than its insistence on the closest attention to the individual. If Roman practice could rely upon stock remedies and patent medicines, Greek practitioners, quite as fully as our own, recognized the paramount importance of dealing with the individual, accord-

---

[10] *Epidem.*, II, iv, 5 (V, 126, Littré); *De locis in homine*, i (VI, 278, Littré). Of course, the Hippocratics would not define the "cause" in the same terms as a modern physician; but doctors, whether ancient or modern, cannot be troubled with the theoretical questions involved in the conception of causation. Their approach is, and must be, practical.

[11] *Epidem.*, I, x (II, 668 f., Littré); *De aere aqua locis, passim.*

ing to the diagnosis resulting from painstaking inquiry and examination of all the factors regarded as significant.[12]

As for the inquiries made, they were of course in the first instance addressed to the patient, provided he was in condition to be questioned.[13] One asked what discomforts or pains he felt, where they were located, and when and under what circumstances they were first experienced. Naturally, one inquired also about his habits and previous condition. The doctor was well aware that the patient's answers were guesses and might be misleading,[14] but one must take account of everything. Most interesting is the fact that inquiries were directed to others besides the patient.[15] This would be inevitable in the cases of very young children and of older persons who might not be able to speak for themselves; but there are other instances also in which the information obtained could not have been given by the patient. Thus the question arises whether gritting the teeth is a new symptom or a habit from childhood,[16] and frequently the habits of patients are inquired into.[17] A boy's navel is said to have been black from birth.[18] Certain effects appearing later proved

[12] A striking exception is to be noted. The Hippocratic treatise *De affectionibus* (VI, 208 ff., Littré), which Galen attributed to Polybus, proposes to instruct the layman in the principles that govern the practice of medicine. It frequently refers to a treatise entitled *Pharmakitis*, apparently a collection of household remedies.
[13] See *De affectionibus*, xxxvii (VI, 246, Littré). See also *Epidem.*, VI, ii, 24 (V, 290, Littré).
[14] *De arte*, xi (VI, 20, Littré).
[15] See Rufus, 208, 11–209, 3, ed. Daremberg.
[16] *Coan praenotions*, ccxxx (V, 634, Littré).
[17] See Fredrich, *Hippokratische Untersuchungen*, pp. 5 f.
[18] *Epidem.*, IV, xxxi (V, 174, Littré).

SCIENTIFIC METHODS 65

that a certain child had had epileptic fits; in such a case, we are told, if one inquires of those who reared him, most will admit the fact, while some will have forgotten or have failed to observe it and will say they know nothing of such an attack.[19] Though the recorded instances are not numerous, they are sufficient to show that this reasonable practice was recognized, and we may be sure that it was observed whenever it seemed desirable.

As has been said, the Hippocratics often mention things that the doctor should note and take account of.[20] One list we may quote because it has been especially cited as exemplary by a noted historian[21] of medicine.

One must note the following: conditions that disappear of their own accord; blisters such as come from fire, where this or that is beneficial or harmful; shapes of parts affected, kinds of motion, swelling, subsidence of swelling, sleep, wakefulness, restlessness, yawning;—lose no time in acting or preventing; vomit, evacuations, spittle, mucus, coughing, belching, swallowing, hiccup, flatulence, urine, sneezing, tears, scratching, plucking or feeling (at hairs or bedding), thirst, hunger, plethora, dreams, pain, absence of pain, the body, the mind, ability to take in one's meaning, memory, voice, persistent silence.[22]

In addition to such indications to be noted by direct observation, the Hippocratics knew there were others hidden to the view. The treatise *On the Art* recognizes that there are hidden ailments and conditions, which

---

[19] *Prorrhetic*, II, x (IX, 30, Littré).
[20] See, for example, *De officina medici*, i (III, 272, Littré); *De victu*, I, ii (VI. 468 f., Littré); and *De morbis*, I, i (VI, 140, Littré).
[21] Haeser, *Lehrbuch der Geschichte der Medicin*, I, 154 f.
[22] *De humoribus*, ii (V, 478, Littré).

nature can and must be compelled to disclose.²³ In respect to diet one tested the degree and tempo of digestibility by causing the patient to disgorge food after a given interval. Other means of exploration or anatomical diagnosis were found in probing wounds. Examination of a man wounded in the loin leads the surgeon to conjecture that death was due to injury to the intestines and the effusion of blood in the abdomen.²⁴ A case of convulsive laughter (*risus sardonicus*) is explained by the assumption that when the arrow was extracted its point remained in the diaphragm.²⁵ In addition to close ocular observation, taste, and smell, the physician resorted to palpation in order to determine location, size, and abnormalities of organs or members; to succussion for the location of congestion;²⁶ and to auscultation in exploring the pleural cavity, lungs, and trachea and particularly in detecting the rasping noises peculiar to pleurisy.²⁷ In this way, doctors contrived a surrogate for the stethoscope and the cardiograph.

One wonders that more attention was not given to the pulse; it has even been asserted that the Hippocratics did not recognize it at all. Such a statement is, however, both in itself incredible and contrary to the evidence.²⁸ However, it is apparently true that Praxagoras, a mem-

²³ *De arte*, xi (VI, 18 ff., Littré).
²⁴ *Epidem.*, V, xxi (V, 220, Littré).
²⁵ *Epidem.*, VII, cxxi (V, 466, Littré).
²⁶ *Coan praenotions*, ccccxxiv (V, 680, Littré); and *De morbis*, I, xv (VI, 164, Littré).
²⁷ *De morbis*, II, lxi (VII, 94, Littré), and III, xvi (VII, 152, Littré).
²⁸ *Prorrhetic*, II, iii (IX, 12, Littré), surely implies feeling the pulse. *De victu*, xlviii (IX, 116, Littré); and Democritus, frag. 120, Diels, mention the pulse.

ber of the Coan school in the generation after Hippocrates, was the first to recognize the importance of the pulse. In respect to diagnosis the merits of the Hippocratics are universally acknowledged, though allowance must, of course, be made for the limitations imposed by the scanty means at their disposal. The celebrated instance of the *facies Hippocratica* is too well known to call for more than mention.

As we have already remarked, the ideal of the Hippocratics aimed at a total unified picture of a diseased state. Their motto might well be the words: "Nothing at random; overlook nothing."[29] In constructing such a picture, however, guided as the Hippocratics were by their rich store of experience in determining what was and what was not significant, they could not fail to observe certain indications that were not typical and consequently suggested differentiation. It was at this point that the school of Cos was distinguished from the Cnidian, which laid great stress on the differences and, consequently, multiplied the names of diseases. It is not for us to judge which school was more in the right; certainly there was good in both tendencies. In the *Epidemics*, especially in Book IV, the special case under consideration is almost always compared with others, and any such comparison must bring out differences as well as similarities.

In any case, a classification presupposed a judgment as to what marks are typical or essential and must, consequently, be founded on experience deemed sufficient. A disease thus described or defined becomes for the physician an entity with a character and presumable course

[29] *Epidem.*, VI, ii, 12 (V, 284, Littré).

that may generally be foreseen. Hence, the Hippocratics regarded their diagnoses as essentially prognoses. They were, however, well aware of the contingent nature of their expectations. Excepting cases in which the indicated outcome was certain death, various possibilities presented themselves. The peccant humor might generally be expected to mature, or be concocted, as a watery rheum seems to change to a glairy mucus, or lymph to pus, and so be eliminated in due course; or it might become encysted in some part, where, unless it was absorbed and thus gradually eliminated, it might cause a local ailment. In either case this was expected to occur at fixed periods known as critical days. It is not important to dwell on the different views among the ancient physicians as to which days were critical, because there was no general agreement on this question, and the periods naturally differed in different diseases. The recognition of crises is not, however, to be so lightly dismissed. A certain periodicity in all things human was from the earliest times perceived by the Greeks and may be said to constitute the very rhythm of life. The ages of man and the relatively fixed periods of gestation of all living beings must have impressed them very deeply. That the doctrine of crises was somehow or other a recognition of the biological character of disease can hardly be questioned; but there is no evidence as to what particular line the Hippocratics took. Assuming the biological nature of the causes of disease, one might suppose that each had its own period of maturation and would thus prepare for its own natural elimination. Whether or not there is a fixed period, there is in many cases a critical stage which the physician awaits with especial anxiety, and upon the way the patient passes it he bases his prognosis. It was not otherwise with the Hippocratics.

In all this there was, of course, a combination of speculation with clinical observation; but may not the same be said of medical theory and practice today? The first impression one gets of Hippocratic medicine is that it was unduly speculative and dogmatic. It cannot be denied that Greek medicine in particular and Greek science in general were of that character. One can easily see why they inevitably became so, when one realizes the limited fund of exact knowledge one commanded. Nevertheless, justice to the pioneers demands that we moderate our too-ready censure by taking account of a fact often overlooked. Greek literature is, perhaps even more than our modern literatures, essentially didactic, and for good or ill teaching it always tends to emphasize the conclusions rather than the processes of thought. Greek medical writings in good part aspired to be accounted literature and were influenced by recognized literary standards even when they were mere jottings for one's personal use, as many a diary in recent times is consciously or unconsciously literary. One's mental habits, the result of education and practice, are not lightly overcome. One who is of the older generation will recall, perhaps with amusement, how science was taught in his youth: principles were enunciated, and at most they were illustrated by examples or by single experiments conducted by the instructor. One recognizes that the inductive method of teaching is a very recent innovation. Knowing that this is true, one will be slow to pass unfavorable judgment on the ancients and conclude that their method was at fault. It was undoubtedly immature, but we have ample grounds for thinking that their spirit was thoroughly scientific.

If general considerations suffice to warn one against hasty judgments unfavorable to the Hippocratics in this regard, a close study of their works affords positive and particular evidence of the way in which they proceeded. A few illustrations drawn from two closely related treatises, *Coan praenotions* and *Prorrhetic*, Book I, will serve our purpose. They are especially instructive because occasionally they refer to the same symptoms. Thus, *Coan praenotions* says: "Cases of delirium that are wild for a short time become violent and announce spasms."[30] But *Prorrhetic* gives: "Cases of delirium that are wild arise from black bile; if they follow menstruation, they are fierce; this often happens. Are the patients taken with spasms? Are cases of speechlessness attended with torpor also due to spasms?"[31] In this instance one treatise states the matter positively, while the other asks a question. Instances occur in which both sources agree in asking questions,[32] evidently because the data available were not deemed sufficient to justify diagnosis or prognosis. This attitude is made clear in cases where the prognosis is introduced by such expressions as "I think so and so will follow"[33] and "I should not be surprised if"[34] or where

[30] *Coan praenotions*, lxxxiv (V, 602, Littré). Cf. *Ibid.*, cli (V, 616, Littré).
[31] *Prorrhetic*, I, cxxiii (V, 552, Littré).
[32] See, for example, *Coan praenotions*, cc (V, 626, Littré); and *Prorrhetic*, I, clxiii (V, 570, Littré).
[33] *Coan praenotions*, xxiv (V, 590, Littré) and clxxxii (V, 622, Littré); and *Prorrhetic*, I, cxlix (V, 564, Littré).
[34] *Coan praenotions*, lxxx (V, 600, Littré).

one author asks a question and the other indicates an expectation. Nothing, it would seem, could better show generalizations in the making; it is as if a modern scholar revealed the steps by which he arrived at conclusions which on occasion he would state dogmatically.

That generalizations, such as those in *Prognostic*, were founded on the minute kind of observations recorded in *Epidemics*, Books I and III, must be obvious to every careful student, though it cannot perhaps be absolutely proved in detail. An instructive instance may be cited from the treatise *De liquidorum usu*. The work as a whole seems clearly to be a very dogmatically phrased extract from a larger treatise no longer extant and therefore admitting no positive judgment regarding its tenor. The statements of the epitome are quite general without any indication of specific evidence for them, except at one point, where the treatment of a young man is reported in detail.[35] This is hardly to be explained except on the assumption that the excerptor found the case so interesting that he could not resist the temptation to copy the statement in full.

There are examples of cautious generalizations, as when we are told, "Those who suffer from coryza and hoarseness, if they have fever, rarely, I believe, have a relapse"[36] or "I have not seen kidney diseases cured in patients over fifty years of age."[37] The same modesty and restraint of statement appears in comments on many

---

[35] *De liquidorum usu*, vi (VI, 134, Littré).
[36] *Epidem.*, VI, iii, 3 (V, 294, Littré).
[37] *Ibid.*, viii, 4 (V, 344, Littré). *Aphorism.*, VI, vi (IV, 564, Littré), says: "Diseases of the kidneys and bladder are hard to cure in the aged."

cases. A certain Simon had eruptions of the skin not attended with much itching. They appeared when he anointed himself near the fire or took a hot bath. "I fancy, if he had taken a Turkish bath, they would have disappeared."[38] Eupolemus had pains in the loin and hip, leading to an ulcer; he was bled in the foot, cauterized, and died. "It seemed likely that if one had made a single, or if need were, two deep incisions, and had removed the pus by the incision,—if this had been done betimes, it seemed likely he would have got well."[39] Similar comments on several other cases are to be found in *Epidemics*, Book V.[40] In view of the uncertain nature of the text tradition, one cannot be certain whether these comments are the reflections of the attending physician, who reviewed his failures, or those of another with other, perhaps wider, experience. No one will fail, however, to approve the temper of such an approach to the physician's task.

The data we have been considering relate to the mental processes of observation and generalization. That they were conducted in a thoroughly scientific spirit is beyond question. Logic, as we understand it, was in the making. Socrates and Plato laid the foundations and Aristotle first erected the structure of formal or deductive logic. Aristotle sketched the outlines of a theory of induction, and the necessary precautions to be observed in inference were more fully elaborated by Skeptics and Empirics, especially by Menodotus, in the first century; but it remained for the most recent times to round out the theory of

[38] *Epidem.*, VI, ii, 15 (V, 284, Littré).
[39] *Ibid.*, V, vii (V, 206, Littré).
[40] See, for examples, cap. xv–xix.

SCIENTIFIC METHODS 73

empirical logic. The Hippocratics, being practical men, observed, judged, and drew conclusions as practical men do today. Obviously, we do not expect to find in them either the conscious need or the practice of the refinements that have resulted from the critical examination of the human faculties. There is, however, ample evidence that they knew and used the essential means of arriving at practically acceptable conclusions. The generalizations they made were founded on minute observation of similarities and differences of cases.

If the Hippocratics did not develop a theory of investigation, they had no doubt reflected on the capacities requisite to successful practice; for they laid emphasis on natural aptitude, early training and education, memory and its purposeful exercise, and diligence.[41] One treatise even offers an account of the intellectual process:

Reason is a sort of memory of data received by sensation; for sensation, being first affected, and reporting objects to the understanding, forms a clear image; and the understanding, receiving the reports repeatedly, noting cause, time, and manner, and storing them in itself, recalls them.[42]

This treatise has been referred to a later date, some scholars even pretending to see in the passage quoted evidence of Stoic or Epicurean influence. Why they should do so is difficult to understand, for there is nothing in it that may not well have been said by any thoughtful Greek at the middle of the fifth century.[43]

[41] *Lex.* ii (IV, 638–40, Littré); and *De arte,* ix (VI, 16, Littré).
[42] Praecepta, i (IX, 250 f., Littré).
[43] See the anonymous *Dialexeis,* ix, Diels; and Plato, *Phaedo,* 96a–b.

One of the works included in the Hippocratic corpus, *De arte,* calls for special mention in this connection. It is a speech dealing with the medical art and appears not to have been written by a physician. Theodor Gomperz thought he could evince his thesis that we owe it to the Sophist Protagoras. Though his suggestion has not found acceptance, there is no reason to doubt that it dates from the fifth century and is therefore contemporary with Hippocrates, if not older. If one attributes it to a Sophist who was not a physician, its significance is actually enhanced; for in that case the knowledge and appreciation of medical practice it displays bears striking testimony not only to the interest in medicine on the part of intelligent laymen but also to their approval of the methods of the profession.

The writer tells us that the art of medicine must be prepared to deal not only with diseases that lie upon the surface and may therefore be detected by the eye but also with those less open to view; for the body has many cavities large and small which may be the seat of distressing ailments.

None of these is visible to the eye, and therefore they are set down as obscure by me and the art; for all their obscurity, however, they have not got the mastery, but have been mastered as far as possible. It is possible to master them, however, so far as the nature of the patients admits of examination and the nature of the investigators is apt at investigation. The discovery is, indeed, made with greater expenditure of pains and time than if it were visible to the eye; what escapes the sight of the eyes is mastered by the sight of the mind, for what the physician cannot see with the eye nor learn by hearing, he pursues with reasoning. He must be careful

SCIENTIFIC METHODS

however to proceed calmly and deliberately rather than with rashness and violence.[44]

Here we have the clearest possible recognition of the process of inferring from the visible and known to the hidden and unknown, which the philosophers of the time emphasized. If due caution was not always observed in arriving at their conclusions, it was not because men of the fifth century had not been warned to fit their theories to the facts rather than facts to their theories. Epicharmus is quoted as bidding one "apply the stone to the yardstick, not the yardstick to the stone"; and of Myson, one of the Seven Sages, it is reported that he used to say that one should not investigate facts by the light of arguments but arguments by the light of facts.[45] This same treatise, *On the Art*, also recognizes that there are ways in which one may subject nature to question and force her, as a slave might be forced on the rack, to yield a secret.[46] The terms "investigation" and "forcing confession" are taken from legal procedures in obtaining evidence by torture, a practice certainly followed before the time of Hippocrates. Scientific terminology and practice were derived from procedures common in daily life, which in the course of time have naturally been refined in law courts as well as in the laboratory. We shall presently have occasion to speak more at length about experimentation and testing.

More fundamental, however, than the practice of testing and experimenting is the process of generalization and

[44] *De arte*, x f. (VI, 16 ff., Littré).
[45] Diogenes Laërtius, I, cviii. Cf. Plutarch, *Moralia*, 75 f. Diogenes Laërtius, II, xxix: "He [Socrates] had the skill to draw his arguments from facts."
[46] Cap. xii (VI, 22 f., Littré).

76　　　　　SCIENTIFIC METHODS

inference. Direct observation—what one sees or hears—is always particular. Generalization proceeds upon the recognition or assumption of similarities, which fall short of identity. Identity, of course, admits of no further inference; hence, the increase of knowledge depends chiefly on the acceptance of inferences from data that present differences as well as similarities. Since most of our thinking is, in the beginning, analogical, how and with what restrictions such inferences can be justified is one of the nicest problems presented to science and philosophy.[47] From the Hippocratics, who were practical men, one will not expect a theoretical discussion and decision of this difficult question; but, in view of their intelligence, one would be surprised if they did not betray a consciousness of the problem and seek to reduce to a minimum the chances of error. Aristotle, of course, states the matter in general terms, saying that experience is the knowledge of the particular, while science or art is the recognition of the general. All practice has to do with the particular; the physician doctors not man in general but the individual, Callias or Socrates, who belongs to the genus Homo. Nevertheless, the best doctor will be he who knows the general, what is good for all men as well as for men of a special character.[48]

The Hippocratics repeatedly emphasize the need of dealing with the individual, but they are also given to generalizations. An especially interesting fact is that they were aware of the problem as it presented itself in their

[47] Aristotle recognized analogical reasoning as a form of induction. Cf. Maier, *Die Syllogistik des Aristoteles*, II, 391 f.
[48] Aristotle, *Metaphysics*, 981a, and *Nicomachean Ethics*, 1180b.

SCIENTIFIC METHODS

practice. Thus, one author[49] says that learning medicine is not like learning to write. You may always write the same characters in the same way, but the doctor must act now so, now otherwise, because at different times and under other circumstances the same treatment will have opposite results. Others[50] insist that individuals differ and that, consequently, the same things are not good for all—one man's poison is another's meat. Still another[51] emphasizes the different reactions of individuals of different constitutions and ages to the same general situations presented by seasons, localities, food, and regimen.

Particularly instructive is a passage in *De articulis* where one is cautioned to exercise care in determining whether or not a joint has been dislocated.[52] The corresponding members are said to be similar in the same individual, though individuals differ greatly one from another. Therefore, one must examine closely the corresponding members of the same person, comparing the healthy member with the one affected, and vice versa. This counsel is, of course, based upon an assumption of fact to which there are many exceptions; but one must bear in mind that Greek doctors and gymnastic trainers had abundant opportunities to observe athletes and to notice the general conformity of the two sides of the body.

Not a little interest attaches to certain analogies assumed or expressly drawn by Hippocratics. Some of

[49] *De locis in homine,* xli (VI, 330 f., Littré).
[50] *De flatibus,* vi (VI, 98, Littré); *De prisca medicina,* xx (I, 622, Littré); and Plato, *Phaedrus,* 271a ff.
[51] *De humoribus,* xvi (V, 496 f., Littré).
[52] Cap. x (IV, 102, Littré).

these will, no doubt, now be regarded as fantastic; but, even so, the significance of these early efforts at understanding should not be overlooked. As has already been pointed out, the range within which comparisons may safely be made had not yet been determined. Although abnormalities and differences between individuals were recognized, they could be discontinued by referring to a standard representing what was "natural" or "for the most part true." A difficulty would arise concerning homologies. They were recognized, as when Empedocles said, "Hair and leaves, and thick feathers of birds, and the scales that grow on mighty limbs are the same thing."[53] No distinction was made, however, between analogies of function and analogies of relation, and there was, of course, no definite notion of the homologous as homogenous, because the similarities were not conceived as due to common descent. It was only the intuition of the poet that enabled him to see resemblance where the man in the street saw none or even emphasized a difference. Perhaps there was more danger in the tacit assumpton of identity between things too far apart; for it is reasonably certain that a number of misconceptions of human anatomy arose from the dissection of lower animals.

Ancient science was, as we have noted, in intention one; modern science has tended to be compartmental, with occasional, though as yet hardly systematic, efforts to break down the partitions and to fill their places with subsidiary or intermediate sciences. The vast domain claimed by human curiosity could not be conquered and

[53] Frag. 82, Diels.

cultivated all at once, despite the valiant and even reckless raids of the early Greeks. Here and there, in widely separated regions, a fair beginning was made, where native faculties sufficed without the aid of elaborate contrivances, the very need of which man did not yet feel. Other fields had perforce to lie fallow until such instruments as the telescope, the spectroscope, the microscope, and the thermometer increased one's range or lent precision to what was vaguely apprehended.

It is true that the Greeks of the fifth century were not wholly unaware of the value of arbitrary, objective standards and units such as modern science requires and employs increasingly in reducing phenomena to forms in which they can be dealt with in definite equations; but the progress was necessarily slow and not uncoördinated. The result was that incipient sciences sprang up here and there, and the successes they attained were hailed and followed up with enthusiasm. To the unimaginative, the findings in these separate fields must have seemed unrelated; but to the eye of genius they displayed points of agreement such as the mind demands in all that it surveys. However mistaken the analogies the Hippocratics noted may have been, their efforts to coördinate what they learned was the index of their scientific endeavor. If the phenomena compared were too far apart, to fill up the gaps between them was a challenge. The problem is not unlike that of instrumental logic in "screwing cause and effect together."

Comparison in the forms of similes and metaphors is one of the essential means not only of lending picturesqueness and vividness to speech but also of making concrete and definite a thought that is hazy and abstract. If the noting of similarities, like the stringing together of like buttons by a child, is the start of bringing order into a chaotic world, the application of clear and distinct ideas, derived from familiar facts and processes, to spheres in which confusion reigns has always been recognized as the beginning of wisdom. That, to judge by the accounts of Plato and Xenophon, was the method of Socrates.[54] What lofty lessons one may draw in this way may be illustrated by Plato's *Gorgias*, in which the medicinal uses of justice are enforced. The discussion in the *Republic* also is essentially a study of justice in the soul of the individual by examining it writ large in the state. No one will fail to recognize the value of such comparisons even in the form of allegory.

The Hippocratics abound in such comparisons; and, though some may be trite or trivial, others not only disclose the range of interests of the physicians and their sense of the unity of all nature but serve to clarify their thinking and to throw light on the problems they sought to explain. Occasionally, a mere collocation reveals an association of ideas that could be justified only by the advance of science. Thus, it is highly suggestive that one finds "food, drink, and breath" mentioned together [55] as nutrients. The Hippocratics commonly regarded respiration chiefly as a means of mitigating and regulating the "inborn heat" of the body; being unaware of the chemical actions that take place in the pulmonary capillaries, they

[54] Maier, *Sokrates*, pp. 180 f., remarks on the similarity in method of Socrates and the medical fraternity.

[55] *De flatibus*, iii (VI, 94, Littré); and *De nutrimento*, xcviii (IX, 118, Littré).

could not know that in breathing we take in essential ingredients and eliminate harmful ones. Yet the association of ideas was not fanciful but prophetic, as one may see by comparing the notion of early Pythagoreans with regard to the respiration of the cosmos and the doctrine of Epicurus that a world can survive only so long as it continues to redress loss of matter by that which it takes in. Obviously, in all these instances the conception arises from the analogy between the cosmos and the microcosm and implies the recognition that breathing is really a form of nutrition.

A most instructive passage occurs in the treatise *Ancient Medicine*.[56] After speaking in the two preceding chapters of the need to study the specific actions of foods on different constitutions and their relations to particular components of the human body, the author proceeds thus:

I maintain that it is also necessary to know which diseased states arise from powers [that is, from properties of foodstuffs] and which from structures. What I mean is roughly that a "power" is an intensity and strength of the humors, while "structures" are the conformations to be found in the human body, some of which are hollow, tapering from wide to narrow; some are expanded; some hard and round; some broad and suspended; some stretched; some long; some close in texture; some loose in texture and fleshy; some spongy and porous. Now, which structure is best adapted to draw and attract to itself fluid from the rest of the body—the hollow and expanded, the hard and round, or the hollow and tapering? I take it that the best adapted is the broad hollow that tapers. One could learn this thoroughly from objects outside the body that can be openly examined. For example, if you

---

[56] Cap. xxii (I, 626 f., Littré).

82   SCIENTIFIC METHODS

open the mouth wide you will draw in no liquid; but if you protrude and contract it, compressing the lips,[57] and then insert a tube, you can easily draw up any liquid you wish. Again, cupping instruments,[58] which are broad and tapering, are so constructed on purpose to draw and attract blood from the flesh. There are many other instruments of a similar nature. Of the parts within the human frame, the bladder, the head, and the womb are of this structure. These obviously attract powerfully, and are always full of liquid from without. Hollow and expanded parts are especially adapted for receiving fluid that has flowed into them, but are not so well suited for attraction. Round solids will neither attract fluid nor receive it when it has flowed onto them, for it would slip round and find no place on which to rest. Spongy, porous parts, like the spleen, lungs, and breasts, will drink up readily what is in contact with them, and these parts especially harden and enlarge on the addition of fluid. They will not be evacuated every day, as are bowels, where the fluid is inside, the bowels enclosing it externally; but when one of these parts drinks up the fluid and takes it to itself, the porous hollows, even the small ones, are everywhere filled, and the soft porous part becomes hard and compact, and neither digests nor discharges. This happens because of the nature of its structure.[59]

It is not necessary to quote the remainder of the discussion of the effects that can be traced to the form or structure of the organs; what is here given suffices to

[57] *De carnibus*, vi (VIII, 592, Littré), refers to sucking with compressed lips. A similar experiment was mentioned by the Ionian philosopher Anaximenes (Diels, V, i, 95, 1 ff.).
[58] The Hippocratics frequently refer to cupping instruments, obviously often used: *Epidem.*, IV, xx (V, 160, Littré); *De locis in homine*, xxii (VI, 314, Littré); *De vulneribus*, xxvii (VI, 430, Littré); *De morbis*, IV, xxxv (VII, 548, Littré); and *De medico*, vii (IX, 212, Littré). Cf. *De carnibus*, vi (VIII, 592, Littré); and Aristotle, *De generatione animalium*, 739b.
[59] Cf. *De locis in homine*, ix (VI, 200 f., Littré).

SCIENTIFIC METHODS

show how this ancient physician endeavored, by the aid of instruments in common use and phenomena to be observed elsewhere, to account for effects produced in the human body with which the practitioner must deal. The reasoning is analogical throughout, and the examples are drawn mostly from physics, though the reference to the sponge introduces an organic product. It is worth while to call attention to this fact, because Littré [60] and others have thought to observe a distinction between the schools of Cos and Cnidus, the school of Cos (represented by Hippocrates) being supposed to seek explanations of physiological matters from biology, whereas the Cnidians had recourse to physics. It is true that most analogies from physics occur in works which presumably show Cnidian influence, but it is impossible, as has already been said, to divide the Hippocratic treatises between the schools. In any case, *Ancient Medicine* bears none of the marks of the Cnidian. On the other hand, there are in works assigned to the Cnidian group numerous instances of biological parallels; hence, we may for our present purposes disregard the distinction.

The fetus is compared to a grain. As the grain on reaching maturity bursts the hull that surrounds it, so the babe in the fullness of time breaks through the chorion and forces its way to the birth.[61] The development of the human embryo is compared with the hatching of hens' eggs [62] or, again, to the growth of a plant from a seed.[63] The formation of embryonic fingers and

[60] *Œuvres complètes d'Hippocrate*, VIII, 7 f.
[61] *De septim. partu*, i (VII, 436, Littré). Cf. *De octom. partu*, xii (VII, 458, Littré). [62] *De natura pueri*, xxix (VII, 530, Littré).
[63] *Ibid.*, xxii (VII, 514, Littré).

toes is likened to the branching of a tree at the end of a limb;[64] and we are told that when the fetus grows and presses on the surrounding organs it squeezes the fat through the caul or omentum, thus producing the milk, just as, if one squeezes a piece of leather soaked in oil, the oil passes through it by osmosis.[65] In like manner, human nutrition and the action of emetics are compared with the process by which a plant draws the needful foodstuffs from the soil.[66] Other analogies drawn from plant life are not uncommon.[67]

We have remarked before that certain mistakes regarding human anatomy were probably due to inferences based on the dissection of lower animals; we may now call attention to two interesting cases in which diseases were explained by observations on animal cadavers. The treatise *On Internal Diseases* expresses the opinion that dropsy often arises from pulmonary ulcers, for its author has seen such ulcers in the lungs of cows, dogs, and swine.[68] He thinks such cases are more frequent in human beings because their diet is less wholesome. The treatise *On Epilepsy* regards that dread disease as a sort of softening of the brain due to flooding and disintegration by phlegm and bases this opinion on a comparison of the brains of sturdied sheep and goats.[69]

[64] *Ibid.*, xix (VII, 506, Littré).
[65] *Ibid.*, xxi (VII, 512, Littré).
[66] *De natura hominis*, vi (VI, 44, Littré); and *De morbis*, IV, xxxiii (VII, 544, Littré).
[67] *De aere aqua locis*, xxiv (II, 92, Littré); *De humoribus*, xi (V, 490, Littré); *De victu*, x (VI, 484, Littré); and *De morbis*, IV, xxxiv (VII, 544, Littré).
[68] Cap. xxiii (VII, 224, Littré).
[69] Cap. xi (VI, 382, Littré).

Whatever one may think of the value of such comparisons, it is obvious that they reveal an honest effort to penetrate the mystery of the unknown by means of the known, or what was assumed to be known and understood. One can hardly blame the pioneers if much that they thought they knew proves to have been partly or wholly mistaken. I recall an extremely interesting address delivered by an eminent scientist years ago, on the advance of science in the preceding quarter century, in which the phrase "we used to think . . . now we know" recurred like a refrain. It would be especially interesting to learn how much that we were then said to know would now have to be introduced by the statement "we used to think."

Analogies drawn from the domain of physics are numerous and sometimes of considerable interest, though others, as in *De victu,* Book I, are either too vague or too fanciful to be significant, except as they reveal the temper of the times. Thus a child in a position that makes delivery difficult is compared to an olive pit placed sideways in the narrow neck of a flask,[70] or the size or abnormal shape of a child is said to be determined by the shape of the mother's womb, as a gourd grown in a flask takes the form of the restricting container or the growth of a plant is curbed by a stone it is forced to evade.[71] Diocles similarly explains the fact that certain rough-edged cuts heal, whereas the smooth surfaces—for example, those of the eyelids, do not grow together, by referring to the difficulty of gluing smooth surfaces to-

---

[70] *De muliebribus,* I, xxxiii (VIII, 78, Littré).
[71] *De semine,* ix-x (VII, 482-84, Littré).

gether, while rough joints adhere very well.[72] As has already been pointed out, there is no difference in principle between such analogies and those which served the purposes of Socrates in his effort to compel his interlocutors to recall philosophy from heaven to earth or to bring nebulous thinking to the test of concrete fact. One recalls the habit of humble folk the world over to reduce every discussion to its lowest terms by summing it up in a proverb. Simple and familiar as this procedure is, it is not to be despised, for it makes for clear thinking and tends to exclude resort to the miraculous.

More significant, however, are those analogies that have to do with fundamental conceptions common to the Hippocratics. From the beginning, Greek science and philosophy were much concerned with heat and cold regarded as distinct opposites. This is perhaps the natural view, but it was perpetuated both by the want of thermometers and by a habit of speech, especially important among the Greeks, who used polar expressions, such as hot and cold, rare and dense, large and small, heavy and light, for want or in lieu of such abstract terms as temperature, density, size, weight. In some cases even the corresponding conception was wanting until appropriate standards and units were accepted. In cosmology the elements were ranged in order of density from earth, through water and air, to fire, and temperature was supposed to correspond exactly to weight. Among the medical fraternity the hot and the cold naturally played an important role, both because of the seasonal changes and, more especially, the association of warmth with life and

[72] *Diocles*, frag. 26, Wellmann.

SCIENTIFIC METHODS

cold with death. Moreover, Greek physicians were most concerned with acute diseases, those marked by high fevers. Consequently one is interested to know how they thought of heat and by what analogies they sought to make its action intelligible.

A fundamental notion was that of the "innate heat" of the body.[73] The body of the living fetus is, of course, warm and derives its heat from the mother.[74] When the child is born it begins to breathe, inhaling air that is cooler than its body. Why it does so is not distinctly stated, but there is no reasonable doubt that the explanation was found in the action of the innate heat. A more detailed account of the process is attributed to Empedocles, though we do not know whether he originated the conception or got it from medical predecessors. According to Aëtius, he held that

The first inspiration of the first animate being came about when the moisture in babes retired and the external air in response to the evacuated part entered into such vessels as were opened. Next, as the innate heat by its outward thrust pressed the air upwards [that is, outwards], expiration resulted, and, by its reciprocating retirement inward affording a reciprocating ingress to the air, inspiration came about.[75]

The rather repetitious statement is based on, or illustrated by, Empedocles' account of the water clock,[76] which may explain the secondary role played by the innate heat. As we have seen, in cosmology temperature

[73] *De victu,* lxii (VI, 576, Littré); and *De morbis,* I, xi (VI, 158, Littré).
[74] *De carnibus,* vi (VIII, 592, Littré); and *De natura pueri,* xii (VII, 486, Littré).
[75] Diels, V, i, 298, 9 ff. See pp. 93–94. [76] Frag. 100, Diels.

was equated with density, and rarefaction and condensation were early conceived as cosmic processes corresponding to growing colder and warmer. Heat liquefies and cold solidifies.[77] The hot tends to be in motion, the cold to remain stationary.[78] Thus the innate heat causes an expansion that must be followed by contraction, drawing air after it. Here we meet an important conception of the Hippocratics, that of "attraction" caused by heat.[79] Motion itself produces heat;[80] whether this fact was explained by referring to friction we are not informed. Heat causes things to move toward it, we are told; the heart, being the warmest part, draws breath (pneuma) from all regions of the body (and obviously also from without), just as, if one lights a lamp or a fire, a current of air will be seen to set toward it, even if there is no draft entering the room from without.[81] The attraction exercised by heat is further illustrated by the phenomenon of the "sun drawing water."[82]

A writer, who agreed with Empedocles and some other "philosophers" in holding that living beings arose spontaneously by putrefaction because of heat and moisture, interested himself also in the process by which membranous integuments were formed.[83] Since he was concerned chiefly with the formation of the veins and entrails, the problem he sought to solve was why the veins, for example, have a relatively hard membranous exterior

[77] *De carnibus*, ix (VIII, 594 f., Littré).   [78] Diels, V, ii, 46, 7.
[79] *De hebdomadibus*, xiv and xix; and Diocles, frag. 16, Wellmann.
[80] *De victu*, II, lxii (VI, 576, Littré).
[81] *De carnibus*, vi (VIII, 592, Littré).
[82] *De natura pueri*, xxv (VII, 522, Littré). See Littré, IX, 278.
[83] *De carnibus*, iii (VIII, 586, Littré).

SCIENTIFIC METHODS

while there is fluid inside them. He also operated mostly with heat and cold, but he regarded the body as composed principally of fatty and glutinous matter produced by putrefaction. The outside of the veins, containing a good deal of cold, was glutinous and by the action of heat was cooked and became membranous, whereas the interior cold, having little fatty or glutinous, melted and turned liquid. He makes it clear, indeed he confesses, that he based his theory on observations made in cooking.[84] In making soup, for example, the heaviest, most glutinous fat rises to the surface and forms a scum that, as it cools, may even be skimmed off in an unbroken sheet. His preoccupation with the tubular veins, hard and obviously colder than the fluid contents, suggests a comparison with the rings, like pneumatic tires, which, according to Anaximander, constituted the celestial bodies: their outside was air or mist, always thought of as cold by the Greeks, while there was inside a mass of fire that showed only at an orifice, like the valve of a tire.[85] Cold, we are told, contracts and solidifies,[86] while heat liquefies and in time dries.[87]

The author of *De carnibus* does not here refer to the influence of cold in forming this tough membrane surrounding the veins, but it is difficult to see how he failed to do so, for in a later discussion he draws attention to

[84] *Ibid.*, iv (VIII, 590, Littré).
[85] Diels, V, i, 83, 33 ff., and 84, 9 ff. Cf. *De morbis*, I, xxvi (VI, 192, Littré).
[86] *De morbis*, I, xxvi (VI, 192, Littré), and IV, lii (VII, 590, Littré); and *De carnibus*, ix (VIII, 596, Littré).
[87] *De carnibus*, ii–iii (VIII, 286–88, Littré); and *De locis in homine*, ix (VI, 292, Littré).

the fact that fresh blood is warm and liquid, but when allowed to cool it coagulates and, if it is not stirred, it is covered by a membrane because of the fibrin it contains.

Proof that the fluid part of the blood is warm is that if you cut any part of the human body, it is warm; but when it is cooled by the cold it contains and the cold outside, a skin and membrane form; and if one removes it and leaves it undisturbed, in a short time another skin will be seen forming. If one continues to remove it, still another skin will form as a result of the cold.[88]

One sees clearly the general conception of these physicians and the phenomena to which they appealed in support of their theories.

In the course of this discussion mention has been made of "attraction," a process that merits further attention. From early times Greek scientists were interested in the phenomena of magnetism and proposed various theories to account for them that we may disregard at present, because their connection with medical views is too remote and a satisfactory discussion would lead us too far afield. The most elaborate theory appears to have been that of Empedocles,[89] and it is also the most interesting for comparison with the views set forth in the Hippocratic writings. It is plain that the latter half of the fifth century was greatly occupied with a group of problems in which interaction between different substances was involved. The formula recurs in *De victu*, Book I: "Carpenters saw wood: one pulls, the other pushes—they accomplish the same result."[90] Attraction or suction es-

---

[88] *De carnibus,* viii–ix (VIII, 594–96, Littré). Cf. Plato, *Timaeus,* 85d
[89] Diels, V, i, 306, 9 ff., and 298, 9 ff.
[90] Cap. vi–vii (VI, 478 ff., Littré).

pecially engaged their attention, and the condition commonly assumed as making suction possible was the existence of a vacuum. They were familiar with the sponge and the cupping glass. Thus Diogenes of Apollonia explained the perception of savors by the moist and spongy texture of the tongue, by which it is able to drink in the juices and pass them along to the sensorium.[91] Fishes, he held, inhale air inclosed in water, drawing it in by the vacuum in the mouth.[92] Even more interesting is his explanation of certain phenomena connected with metals. To understand his reasoning, it is essential to bear in mind that metals in the form they were ordinarily used had been smelted and had been in a liquid state and that all liquids were thought of as water or closely analogous to water. Did not water, also, when frozen become solid? So Diogenes held that when bronze or iron rust when placed in the fire they lose moisture, or, if covered with vinegar, the acid draws moisture from them. In the former case it was, for him, an example of the attraction exerted by fire; in the latter probably a supposed affinity of water for acid, as of moisture for salt.[93]

The existence of vacua in the human body accounted for many things. The softer flesh of women, compared with that of men, was supposed to be due to its greater porosity. This notion underlies a good deal of the gynecology of the Hippocratics.[94] Thus fat women were sup-

[91] Diels, V, ii, 57, 8 ff.
[92] *Ibid.*, 58, 13 ff. Cf. *De flatibus*, iii (VI, 94, Littré).
[93] Diels, V, ii, 58, 22 ff.
[94] Cf. *De sterilibus mulieribus, passim* (VIII, 408 ff., Littré); *De muliebribus*, xxiv (VIII, 64 f., Littré); and Aristotle, *De generatione animalium*, 747a.

posed to be incapable of conceiving, because the veins of their wombs are stopped, conception being thought of as a form of suction. The means employed to promote conception were, in good part, aerating and drying the organs by fumigations, and the tests applied to determine whether the woman was in condition to conceive were of the same kind. We are told that if on the following morning she smells or tastes, or if her hair gives off, the odor of a vaginal pessary inserted the previous evening, she may expect to have her hopes fulfilled.[95] In any case, it appears, there was supposed to be involved the attraction of heat, whether produced by fumigation or by pungent substances in the pessary. Aristotle has the same process in mind:

> The womb because it is warm attracts the semen; and the efflux and concentration of the menses cause inflammation in that organ, so that it attracts, just as conic[96] vessels, after having been rinsed with hot liquid, suck up water when the inverted mouth is immersed in it.[97]

The philosophers differed among themselves on the question whether a vacuum really existed. As we have seen, Empedocles and Anaxagoras experimented with inflated bags and showed that the container, regarded as empty because it contained only air, was, nevertheless, not really empty. The medical fraternity appear, however, to have had no doubt of the existence of an actual vacuum and based many of their theories upon it. Like the Ionians, who emphasized the contrasting states of

---

[95] *De sterilibus mulieribus*, ccxiv (VIII, 416, Littré).
[96] The reading, evidently right, proposed by Platt.
[97] *De generatione animalium*, 739b.

rarefaction and condensation, they could not account for physiological processes except on the supposition that what appeared to be full might have empty interstices capable of admitting another substance. Thus, how was one to account for growth from within and nutrition, if the seemingly solid body did not have "pores" within it, by which the added materials could be received and distributed? Leucippus, apparently, drew attention to the familiar instance, formerly to be witnessed on every farm, of the ash barrel that (as he thought) could take up just as much water as if it contained no ashes.[98]

In any case, whether one accepted an actual void or not, there must be some way, like the circular displacement of Aristotle, of providing for a substance yielding before another, for "everything flows into what makes place before it."[99] More definitely the yielding was understood to be due to a partial or total vacuum. This might be produced by suction, as in the flow of milk to the mother's breast,[100] or to the motion of a humor caused by heat drawing some other fluid after it.[101] The principle of the *horror vacui,* or, as Erasistratus called it, "the pursuit of the evacuated," was thoroughly familiar to the Hippocratics.[102] Indeed, the theory of the circulation of the fluids of the body, that accounts for both health and disease, and of respiration, in which the innate heat and the cold air inhaled in respiration alter-

[98] Diels, V, ii, 76, 31 ff. Cf. [Aristotle], *Problem.,* 938b.
[99] *De locis in homine,* ix (VI, 292, Littré).
[100] *De natura pueri,* xxi (VII, 514, Littré).
[101] *De muliebribus,* I, xvi (VIII, 54, Littré).
[102] *De victu,* II, lxiv (VI, 578, Littré); *De morbis,* IV, xl (VII, 560, Littré); and *De natura pueri,* xxi (VII, 512, Littré). See pp. 87-88.

nately retreat and pursue each other, is founded on this conception.

The principal organs, conceived as reservoirs of the humors, were thought of as related in the same way as vessels connected by communicating tubes, so that if a fluid was taken from one reservoir it was replaced by another humor following hard upon the one withdrawn.[103] Analogously, the phenomena were explained by the example of "water on a table,"[104] referring to the familiar fact that water, because of surface tension, may stand on a table above the level surface, but will flow off once a wet streak is made to its edge and it is set in motion. Several passages already mentioned contain references to the action of sponges or small veins and the way in which they attract moisture—in a word, to what we now regard as surface tension or capillarity. We do not know who first utilized these phenomena in explaining processes not so familiar, but it is probable that more than one man of science had recourse to them.

A particularly interesting example is Diogenes of Apollonia, who sought to explain the (to the Greeks) paradoxical floods of the Nile. Seneca gives the account of his attempt:

The sun draws moisture to itself; the earth derives its moisture from the sea and then from other waters. It is impossible that one land be dry while another overflows, for all parts are pierced through and permit moisture to circulate, and so the dry derive it from the wet; otherwise, if it did not receive any, the earth would dry out. Consequently the sun

---

[103] *De morbis*, IV, xxxix (VII, 556 f., Littré).
[104] *Ibid.*, li (VII, 588 f., Littré); and *De natura pueri*, xviii (VII, 502, Littré).

SCIENTIFIC METHODS

attracts moisture from all quarters, but most of all from those it most assails—the southern. The more a land dries out, the more moisture it attracts; as, in lamps, the oil flows to the point where it is consumed by the flame, so water tends to the point where the force of the heat and the burning earth call it. Whence then does it draw it? From the quarters where winter always reigns—the northern regions overflow. That is why the Black Sea constantly flows with a strong current into the Mediterranean, always in one direction. . . . The sun bakes Egypt more; therefore the Nile has a higher flood.[105]

If in some of these analogies one sees inferences drawn from such familiar instruments as the tube (or straw) for drawing liquid from a container, to the cupping glass, in common use among doctors, or to the water clock by which pleaders in court found their allotted time determined, these were by no means the only mechanical devices so employed. The effect on the humors of a person afflicted by a disease produced by unfavorable weather is compared to that to be observed in a Scythian churn;[106] and a humor, prevented by pressure of accumulated blood from flowing, is said to resemble a liquid in a narrow-necked flask held back by air closing the opening. Once it begins to flow, however, all will run off.[107] The philosophers had made similar comparisons, as, for example, Empedocles likened the eye to a lantern[108] and the ear to a bell or trumpet.[109] The latter analogy recalls that of Archytas,[110] who said that sounds too loud cannot enter our hearing just as narrow-necked vessels admit nothing

[105] *Naturales quaestiones*, IV, ii.
[106] *De morbis*, IV, li (VII, 584, Littré).
[107] *Ibid.* (VII, 588, Littré).
[108] Frag. 84, Diels.
[109] Frag. 99, Diels.
[110] Frag. 1, Diels.

if one tries to pour in a great quantity of liquor at once. Aristotle himself was not above illustrating earthquakes by referring to the pulsation, quivering, and palpitation of the living body.[111] Indeed in his *Meteorologica*, quite regularly and in *De caelo* frequently, he relied on physiological analogies in seeking to explain phenomena in physics. Like the philosophers, the Hippocratics referred to the phenomena of the segregation of like to like by a vortex motion,[112] and we find the formation of calculi in the bladder compared to the smelting of ore when the metal collects and solidifies.[113] More interesting, perhaps, are the parallels drawn between sweat and the condensing steam on a kettle lid and the explanation of yawning as due to the pressure of gas in the stomach, as the pressure of steam in a boiling kettle lifts the lid.[114]

It hardly needs to be said that many of the observations just mentioned as instances of analogical reasoning might almost, if not quite, as well be set down as the result of experimentation, for it is not always easy or even possible to distinguish. The conclusion drawn from an experiment will henceforth be accepted as a fact that may at any time be cited by way of illustration in confirmation of other observations and the inferences to which they point. Ignoring this fact and carelessly accepting certain dicta of supposed authorities, many modern writers have declared that the Greeks were not in the

---

[111] *Meteorologica*, 366b.

[112] *De morbis*, IV, lv (VII, 600, Littré); and *De natura pueri*, xvii (VII, 498, Littré).

[113] *De morbis*, IV, lv (VII, 600, Littré). Cf. *De aere aqua locis*, ix (II, 38, Littré).

[114] *De flatibus*, viii (VI, 102 f., Littré).

habit of experimenting or that, if and when they did, it was solely in the interest of confirming conclusions arrived at by abstract reasoning. Thus Bacon, in the *Novum organum*,[115] asserted that we should give no weight to the fact that Aristotle in some of his works was concerned with experiments, because he had formed his conclusions before and made experiments conform with what he wished. In another connection Bacon referred, obviously as confirmatory evidence for his contention, to the circumstance that Aristotle cited very few authorities and when he did so that he mentioned them only in order to refute or differ from them.

We shall presently have to consider more at length the question of the scientific value and the limitations of experimentation among the Greeks, but it is important, because of the weight still given to Bacon's opinions, to inquire whether he was a competent judge. One need not quarrel with him about Aristotle, whose works he had studied, though even there exception must be taken. Whewell, also, being like Bacon chiefly interested in Aristotle, took much the same view. The first objection to urge against these much quoted authorities is that neither had a first hand knowledge of the older scientific writings of the Greeks except those of Plato and Aristotle. That is, however, a minor point. Of far greater importance is the obvious fact that Bacon knew little of the way the human mind actually works and had not reflected on the difference between arriving at conclusions and presenting them for the acceptance of others.

Psychologists have sufficiently emphasized the proc-

[115] Aphorism No. 63.

esses by which one passes from direct observation of particulars to generalizations by noting similarities and differences, classifying and forming hypotheses which are tested and modified by experience; and they have shown that one proceeds experimentally throughout. What makes possible so crude a view as that implied by Bacon's statement is the fact that the mind commonly functions automatically, as it were, and that in consequence we are generally unaware of the steps it has taken in the march to its goal. Every scholar or scientist can bear witness to this; for, unless he has kept a minute dated record of his investigations, he will not be able to give a true account of the way he arrived at his conclusions. And it is no less obvious that one cannot judge by the form of exposition what labor of the mind has gone into a seemingly dogmatic or a priori pronouncement.

This is especially true of all writing that aspires to be literature; for, as among the ancient Greeks, it has never been the fashion among literary men to multiply footnotes and to display the scaffolding of the structure; that is the way of the grammarian and the scholar who writes for scholars. Few of these have the courage or the presumption of a Wilamowitz, who could declare that competent scholars would, of course, know the evidence on which his conclusions rested and that no one else was entitled to pass judgment upon them.

Nevertheless, no one, not even a scholar, actually pretends to give a full account of his studies. Moret quotes from Maspero, the eminent Egyptologist, a statement that might well have been made by any great scholar, ancient or modern:

SCIENTIFIC METHODS

I have never dreamed of boring the public with the amount of toil I have had to undertake before arriving at the point I have attained. Nineteen twentieths remains in my hands, and for the most part I have published results only, without indicating the procedures employed in obtaining them.[116]

Can one conceive of Aristotle carrying in his head the innumerable details regarding animals presupposed by the statements of fact in his zoological treatises? Yet there remain no notebooks of his. Of the experiments of Roger Bacon and of Boyle and his associates there is no record.[117] Especially among the Greeks, who tended to make literature of all they wrote, rough notes, assuming as a matter of course that in many instances they must have been made, were little likely to survive. I cannot do better than quote what I have elsewhere written:

The elaborate structure of evidence which the scholar or scientist erects is only the scaffolding of the artisan, extremely useful in the completion of his edifice, but distracting and offensive to the artist, who prefers to contemplate the whole, defined only by the harmonious lines that give it character and meaning. A science is essentially a work of art, and the satisfaction one derives from a survey of it is essentially aesthetic. Stripped of the scaffolding, it suggests nothing of the toil that went to the making of it. The impression it leaves on the mind is much the same as that made by the great pyramid of Egypt on the Greek historian: "Most wonderful of all, though preparatory works of such magnitude were constructed in the desert, not a trace remains of the ramp nor of the working of the stones, insomuch that one might fancy that it was not builded bit by bit by the labor of men, but was set down by some god as a completed structure all at once

---

[116] *Revue de l'histoire des religions*, LXXIV, 274.
[117] Allbutt, *Greek Medicine in Rome*, p. 509.

100 SCIENTIFIC METHODS

in the surrounding sands."[118] The historian of science needs to have some knowledge of the working of the mind, and he requires no less something of the imagination of this Greek historian.[119]

As we have said, it is often difficult or impossible to distinguish in a record between an observation mentioned by way of analogy and an experiment purposely made to illustrate a case. As the mind naturally passes from similar to similar and only afterwards justifies its inference, so the scholar or scientist, whether aware of it or not, commonly leaps to the formulation of a question or to a tentative hypothesis on the basis of a preliminary survey of data only partially known, in which, however, he perceives enough resemblance to suggest further inquiry. Whether or not the search is prosecuted to the point of demonstration depends on many factors, some of which are individual and personal, others more general, such as the temper of the times and the social milieu. We have had occasion to mention experiments made by the philosophers Empedocles and Anaxagoras and explorations, equivalent to experiments, undertaken by the physician Alcmaeon. We shall now have to consider some further instances of similar procedures by the Hippocratics and to estimate their value from the point of view of methodology. It need hardly be said that they leave much to be desired, though they manifest a truly scientific spirit. Just why the Hippocratics fell, or seem to have fallen, short of the desirable perfection of method one cannot say; certainly their failure, real or apparent, cannot be

[118] Diodorus Siculus, I, lxiii, 7.
[119] *The Heroic Age of Science*, pp. 79 f.

SCIENTIFIC METHODS

charged solely to the character of the available record, nor can it be said to be due wholly to ignorance of the necessary safeguards to be observed in experimenting.

This conclusion, if not proved, is certainly suggested by the example of Herodotus, a historian who wrote in the latter half of the fifth century and who was, therefore, contemporary with the older Hippocratics. He is of special importance as a witness because, despite his charm as a writer and his keen interest in every phase of life, his want of understanding of contemporary science is such that he cannot be regarded as representing the best thought of his time. In the second book of his history he mentions several experiments. He twice refers to the use of the sounding line, once to confirm his view that Egypt (the flood plain of the Nile) is alluvial, silt brought by the river from Ethiopia,[120] as is proved by soundings in the Mediterranean and the projection of the Delta beyond the general trend of the coastline. The other case is of sufficient interest to justify going more into detail.

Regarding the sources of the Nile, none of the Egyptians, Libyans, or Greeks, with whom I conversed, professed to have knowledge, except the secretary of the temple of Athena in the Egyptian city of Sais; and he seemed to me to be jesting when he claimed to have exact knowledge. What he said was this, that between the city of Syene in the Thebaid and Elephantine there are two mountains rising to sharp peaks, called respectively Crophi and Mophi, and that the springs of the Nile, which are bottomless, flow from between these mountains, half the water flowing northward to Egypt, half southward to Ethiopia. That the springs are bottomless, he said, Psammetichus, King of Egypt, showed by experiment; for

---
[120] Herodotus, II, x.

though he let down a rope of many thousand fathoms' length he could not reach bottom. Thus if the secretary told the truth about the experiment it only proved, I think, that there are strong eddies there and an upward rush of water such that, as the water strikes the mountains, the line let down can not reach the bottom.[121]

Herodotus plainly recognized that the experiment, if made, did not prove what it was supposed to prove.

Much more significant is still another tale he tells.

The Egyptians before the reign of Psammetichus regarded themselves as the oldest people of all mankind; but since that king, upon ascending the throne, conceived a desire to know who were the oldest people, they believe that the Phrygians are older than themselves, but that they themselves are older than all others. Now Psammetichus, not being able by inquiry to discover any means to that end, contrived the following scheme. He took two boys at random and gave them to a herdsman to bring them up among his flocks, after the following manner. He commanded that no one should utter any word in their presence, but that they should lie by themselves in a lonely hut. The herdsman was to lead in goats at the proper times, give the children their fill of milk, and do all else that was needful; this Psammetichus did and ordained, desiring to hear what word the children would first utter, once they passed beyond unintelligible babbling. And so it befell; for, after the herdsman had for two years observed these instructions, as he opened the door and entered, both the children ran to him with outstretched hands and cried "becos." At first the herdsman, on hearing this, held his tongue; but when, as he came often and cared for the children, he observed that that word was frequently spoken, he made it known to his master, and at his bidding brought the children into the king's presence. And now that he himself had heard, Psammetichus set

---

[121] Herodotus, II, xxviii.

SCIENTIFIC METHODS

about inquiring what people used the word "becos" to signify something, and he learned that the Phrygians so called bread. Thus, and upon such evidence, the Egyptians conceded that the Phrygians were older than they. This version of the story I heard from the priests of Hephaestus at Memphis. Certain Greeks, among other foolish tales, relate that Psammetichus cut out women's tongues and had the children brought up among them.[122]

It is hardly necessary to point out here, what I have tried to show elsewhere,[123] that this is a satirical skit of a clever Greek—not Herodotus—on the Egyptian pretensions of extreme antiquity. What concerns us at present is the light the tale throws on experimentation as conceived by the Greeks of the fifth century B.C., or, if I am right in my contention that the tale was derived from Hecataeus of Miletus, of the sixth century. It is plain, at first sight, that we have here an experiment in due form, conducted according to precise specifications with the intention of excluding everything that might vitiate the result. Furthermore, the herdsman is not content with hearing the word spoken once, but waits to see whether it is regularly repeated; finally, the king, not satisfied with report, himself confirms the findings of his assistant. If the experiment failed to establish the point it was to determine, it was because of an oversight—failure to realize that the children learned speech by imitation and therefore did their best to reproduce the bleating of their nurses, the goats.

[122] Herodotus, II, iii.
[123] "Hecataeus and the Egyptian Priests in Herodotus, Book II," *Memoirs of the American Academy of Arts and Sciences*, XVIII (1935), 58 ff.

Obviously, though Herodotus betrays no recognition of the fact, the wag from whom he borrowed the tale was fully aware of the omission. He was even malicious enough to suggest that while the herdsman might be trusted to hold his tongue in order to insure the success of the experiment, it would be necessary, if women were to be employed, to cut out their tongues. In any case it is evident that one was not unaware that meticulous care must be exercised in order to insure against failure or arriving at ridiculous conclusions.

While it is obvious, therefore, that one had given thought to the need of precautions and the refinement of the technique of experimentation, it is equally plain from mistaken results that practice must have failed to keep pace with theory. That experimentation was widely practiced is, however, obvious, especially because in this case it is clearly travestied. One does not burlesque a practice unless it has become familiar. If the tale dates, as I believe, from the sixth century, it is significant; in the fifth century, as our account shows, every one, especially men of science, appears to have engaged in the sport, in so much that it could be treated as a fad. In the *Clouds* of Aristophanes, produced in 423 B.C., Socrates and his associates are represented as a philosophical school engaged in typical pursuits, and everything they do is, of course, turned to ridicule. That is what lends significance to the jibe that Socrates set his pupils the problem to find out how far, measured by its own feet, a flea would jump [124]—a neat problem in mathematics.

An interesting experiment is suggested in the Hippo-

[124] Vs. 144.

SCIENTIFIC METHODS 105

cratic treatise *On the Heart*. It purports to prove that when one drinks, a certain quantity of liquid finds its way into the lungs.

The greater part of what a man drinks passes into the stomach, for the gullet is like a funnel and receives whatever we swallow; but a very small part, so small as not to be noticed, passes through the opening into the windpipe, for the epiglottis is an accurate cover and will not let anything more than a liquid pass through. Here you have the proof: If you mix water with a blue or red pigment and give it to a very thirsty animal—preferably a pig, for the brute is neither nice nor squeamish—and if you then, while it is still drinking, cut its throat, you will find the windpipe discolored. But the experiment calls for an expert.[125]

One will not fail to observe the care recommended in performing the operation. The pig must be very thirsty, to make sure that it will gulp down the water greedily, evidently because one had noticed that one readily chokes by getting some water in the windpipe under such circumstances, and the throat must be cut while the brute is still drinking, and cut by an expert, to insure a quick clean operation. Of course, even so, one could hardly avoid having the pig squeal and draw in breath while there was water in its mouth. That was overlooked. The use of pigments to enable one to trace the water was ingenious and reminds one of the means adopted in testing the adjustment of pistons in an internal combustion engine. Despite the care exercised, the experiment led to a false inference.

[125] Cap. viii (IX, 84 f., Littré). The notion that part of the liquid we drink reaches the lungs is also expressed in cap. i (IX, 80, Littré) and in *De natura ossium*, xiii (IX, 186, Littré).

Hardly less interesting than the experiment is, however, the discussion of the inference from it by the author of *De morbis*, Book IV.[126] He tells us that many accept it as true, and after marshaling a long array of arguments—some of considerable interest on their own account—to disprove it, he adds:

> This is my proof, and what is more, I should not have adduced any such evidence for my conclusion but for the fact that many men believe that drink goes to the lungs, and that it is necessary to bring many proofs against beliefs strongly held, if one is to convert an unwilling opponent from his former opinion by one's arguments.

The false view, held also by Plato,[127] we learn from Plutarch and Aulus Gellius, was finally disposed of by the anatomical researches of Erasistratus.[128]

So far as food and drink are concerned the procedure of the physicians was necessarily experimental.[129] It is worth while to quote a passage from *Ancient Medicine* to show how well aware the Hippocratics were of this fact.

> The art of medicine would never have been discovered to begin with, nor would any medical research have been conducted—for there would have been no need for medicine—if sick men had profited by the same mode of living and regimen as the food, drink and mode of living of men in health, and if there had been no other things for the sick better than these. But the fact is that sheer necessity has caused men to seek and to find medicine, because sick men did not. and do not, profit by the same regimen as do men in health. To trace

---

[126] Cap. lvi (VII, 604–8, Littré).
[127] *Timaeus*, 70c ff. and 91a.
[128] Plutarch, *Convivium*, 698a; and Aulus Gellius, XVII, xi. Cf. Philistion, frag. 7, Wellmann.
[129] See Diodorus Siculus, I, xliii, 1.

the matter still further back, I hold that not even the mode of living and nourishment enjoyed at the present time by men in health would have been discovered, had a man been satisfied with the same food and drink as satisfy an ox, a horse, and every animal save man, for example, the products of the earth—fruits, wood, and grass. For on these they are nourished, grow, and live without pain, having no need at all of any other kind of living. Yet I am of opinion that to begin with man also used this sort of nourishment.[130] Our present ways of living have, I think, been discovered and elaborated during a long period of time. For many and terrible were the sufferings of men from strong and brutish living when they partook of crude foods, uncompounded and possessing strong powers [qualities]—the same in fact as men would suffer at the present day, falling into violent pains and diseases quickly followed by death. Formerly indeed they probably suffered less, because they were used to it, but they suffered severely even then. The majority naturally perished, having too weak a constitution, while the stronger resisted longer, just as at the present time some men easily deal with strong foods, while others do so only with severe pains. For this reason the ancients too seem to me to have sought for nourishment that harmonized with their constitution, and to have discovered that which we use now. So from wheat, after steeping it, winnowing, grinding and sifting, kneading and baking, they produced bread, and from barley they produced cake. Experimenting with food they boiled or baked, after mixing, many other things, combining the strong and uncompounded with the weaker components so as to adapt all to the constitution and power of man, thinking that from foods which, being too

---

[130] Every indication suggests that our author here echoes an early discussion of the origin of civilization and that civilization was represented as first arising in Egypt, as the entire tenor of Herodotus, Book II, implies. It is, however, evident that Herodotus did not originate the theory, and the later tradition obviously goes back to an account earlier and less fragmentary than his. Upon that earlier source depend Plato, *Critias*, 115b ff.; and Diodorus Siculus, I, xliii.

strong, the human constitution cannot assimilate when eaten, will come pain, disease, and death, while from such as can be assimilated will come nourishment, growth, and health. To this discovery and research what juster or more appropriate name could be given than medicine, seeing that it has been discovered with a view to the health, saving, and nourishment of man, in the place of that mode of living from which came the pain, disease, and death? [131]

The interest in the advancement of knowledge here displayed was nothing new, though it was especially cultivated by the Sophists of the latter half of the fifth century. Xenophanes had already emphasized the gradual accumulation and extension of knowledge and the historians, beginning in the sixth century, had sought to ascertain the sources of useful inventions. Dramatists, embellishing old myths and legends, represented the Greek culture-heroes Prometheus and Palamedes as the rivals of the culture-gods, Triptolemus and Dionysus, or Osiris and Isis, in inventing and spreading the knowledge of the arts. One of the so-called cyclical poets, probably in the *Sack of Troy*,[132] seems to have first distinguished between surgery and internal medicine in relating that Poseidon conferred these gifts upon his sons, making Podaleirius a surgeon and Machaon a physician endowed with knowledge of hidden disorders (so that he recognized the madness of Ajax by the flashing of his eyes) and the power to heal them. The notion that necessity is the mother of

---

[131] Cap. iii (I, 574 f., Littré), tr. Jones. E. Chauvet, *La Philosophie des médecins grecs*, p. 41, well characterizes this treatise. In spirit and method it seems to me to bear a strong resemblance to the history of Thucydides.
[132] *Iliupersis*, frag. 5.

SCIENTIFIC METHODS 109

invention, too, was nothing new,[133] though short-sighted scholars have imagined that it originated with Protagoras or Democritus.

Were our knowledge of fifth-century thought less fragmentary, we should find, I am sure, that there were current all the important ideas that took various elaborated forms in the works of Plato and Aristotle, who drew their inspiration from earlier sources. It was natural in a period that witnessed so extraordinary a burst of enthusiasm for science that, while one imagined that knowledge was either already complete or just on the point of attaining perfection, it should be suggested that the progress achieved was entirely due to the application of the right method and owed nothing to chance.[134]

Sober reflection, however, compelled one to recognize the value of luck, and to see that, whether or not one acknowledged the existence of chance,[135] there followed from what the physician did many a result, good and bad, neither intended nor foreseen.[136] All the elements

---

[133] It is clearly implied in Sophocles, *Oedipus rex*, 44 f., where the text is evidently corrupt. The required meaning is that disaster (that is, stern necessity) spurs one to find a remedy.

[134] *De prisca medicina*, xii (I, 598, Littré).

[135] *De arte*, vi (VI, 10, Littré), insists that the so-called "spontaneous," what occurs without cause or by chance, is not a reality but a mere name.

[136] *De morbis*, I, vi–viii (VI, 154 ff., Littré), enlarges upon things the physician may do by chance or unintentionally that help or harm his patient, for many things "just happen." *De affectionibus*, xlv (VI, 254, Littré), says: "It is all-important to know medicaments given as potions and applied to wounds; for they are not intentionally discovered by men but rather by chance, nor by professionals rather than by laymen." Plutarch (Diels, V, i, 379, 15 ff.) quotes Ion of Chios as saying that chance, though differing widely from wisdom, yet achieves similar results.

were thus present for the debate among philosophers whether chance should be admitted to have real existence. One suspects that Socrates, if he held the beliefs imputed to him by Plato, would have solved the problem on the principles set forth in the *Gorgias*, that is to say, on the distinction between willing or wishing, between one's ultimate purpose and the immediate objective.

As we have seen, respiration was understood to be a kind of nutrition, and as the necessary condition of life it naturally occupied an important place in the thought of the Hippocratics. In the preceding discussion we have repeatedly had occasion to speak of it from different points of view; but there are still other aspects that may profitably be considered. From the earliest times, one imagines, men must have wondered at the difference between men and fish, men living in the air, fish in water and in sea water at that. Heraclitus, illustrating his principle of relativity, had said: "The sea is the purest and the most abominable water; for fishes potable and wholesome, for men undrinkable and deadly."[137] How could that be? According to Aelian,[138] Democritus, followed by Aristotle[139] and Theophrastus, contended that there was fresh water contained in the sea, and it was this that fish live on. Aristotle suggests an experiment to prove this, which must have been generally accepted on other grounds, such as the observation that when sea water evaporates salt remains, whereas the vapor, when it con-

---

[137] Frag. 61, Diels.
[138] *Hist. animal.*, IX, lxiv.
[139] Aristotle, *Historia animalium*, 590a; and *Meteorologica*, 355a and 358a–b.

SCIENTIFIC METHODS 111

denses and falls in rain, is shown to be sweet.[140] But fish certainly must breathe, since they are living creatures. The solution is found in the assumption that water contains air, and that it is thus that they breathe. It is not necessary to go into Aristotle's views, except to say that he had personally made, or knew of, experiments with frogs and tortoises to see whether, when they are drowned, air bubbles rise to the surface, and that he knew that when fish die this is not the case.[141]

How much experimenting along this line had gone before we do not know, but it is hardly possible that there was none. Aristotle reports:

Democritus of Abdera and certain other writers on the subject of respiration have not spoken particularly of the bloodless animals last mentioned, but they seem to assert that all animals breathe. Anaxagoras, however, and Diogenes say that all animals respire, and they maintain that fishes and oysters have a sort of respiration. Anaxagoras declares that when fishes discharge water through their gills they inhale the air that is developed in the mouth and so respire. Diogenes, on the other hand, says that when fishes discharge water through their gills they inhale air, by the action of the vacuum formed in the mouth, out of water that surrounds the mouth, on the theory that water contains air.[142]

Evaporation was, of course, a familiar fact and was commonly regarded as the conversion of water into air, when its volume is increased and may break its container.[143] A slightly different view is expressed in *De morbis*, Book IV:

[140] *Meteorologica*, 358b, shows that Aristotle had experimented.
[141] *De respiratione*, 471b.
[142] *Ibid.*, 470b.
[143] Aristotle, *De caelo*, 305b.

If one does not apply the proper remedies to a fever arising from all the moisture, the disease will spread, so far as it masters the humors, in this wise: as the body grows hot the dropsical humor evaporates through it, as being most inimical to fire, and there remains the fatty and the soft, that is the bilious, which serves most as nutriment to the fire. It evaporates on this wise: if one pours water and oil into a vessel and places a big wood-fire under it for a long time, the water will be much less in quantity, for it will evaporate from the vessel, whereas the oil will be but little less, because the water by reason of its rarefied nature can be subtilized by the fire and, becoming light, evaporate, whereas the oil, cohering with itself and being dense, cannot be subtilized nor evaporate the same as water.[144]

Here it seems to be implied that evaporation is due to the escape of contained air from the interstices of the rarefied water.

Water was boiled not only in cooking but also for the purpose of purifying it,[145] and various things were obviously boiled solely for the purpose of discovering what effect was produced by the operation. One must not forget that evaporation was regarded as exhalation, that is as respiration, as is abundantly shown by the theories regarding the origin of winds from the upward current of air attending the formation of mist or fog by streams and melting snow or ice. In this connection, one should recall the association of warmth with gentle and of cold with strong winds and of the experiment imputed to Anaximenes,[146] who thought breath exhaled gently from the wide-open mouth was warm, while that blown from

---

[144] Cap. xlix (VII, 580, Littré).
[145] *De aere aqua locis*, viii (II, 36, Littré).
[146] Diels, V, i, 95, 3 ff.

SCIENTIFIC METHODS

compressed lips was cold. The apparent effect, we know, is due to evaporation. Much the same facts underlie the observations that in hot weather one sweats in the shade or when covered but not in the sun or when uncovered.[147] Experience, if not experiment, accounts for such observations, as also for the realization that fanning oneself postpones and intensifies the sensation of heat instead of relieving it.[148]

The Hippocratics mention two experiments connected with evaporation. One has to do with capillarity; if one suspends over water for two days and nights loose pure wool and a pure woolen fabric closely woven, of the same weight, one will find on weighing them that the former is much the heavier, because it absorbs far more of the water vapor.[149] The other concerns the direct transition from the solid to the gaseous state: if in winter one pours a measured quantity of water into a vessel and sets it out of doors where it will freeze quickly and on the morrow brings it into a warm room where it will melt as quickly as possible, one will find on measuring it that the quantity is considerably reduced.[150] It was very well known to the Hippocratics that different waters had different weights,[151] and it had long been a question debated among men of science why the sea is salt, the favorite theory being that the salt content, which is eliminated by

---

[147] *De aere aqua locis*, viii (II, 34, Littré).
[148] [Aristotle], *Problem.*, 967a.
[149] *De muliebribus*, I, i (VIII, 12, Littré).
[150] *De aere aqua locis*, viii (II, 36, Littré).
[151] *Ibid.*, i (II, 12, Littré); *Aphorism.*, V, xxvi (IV, 542, Littré); Aristotle, *Meteorologica*, 355b and 359a; and Theophrastus, frag. 159, Wimmer.

evaporation, derives from the earth through which it filters. In proof of this conclusion, one referred to the existence of salt mines and the efflorescence of soda (for example, in Egypt).

One might add many other examples of observations derived from experiments, whether made in the ordinary routine of life or in the practice of the industrial arts. That relatively few can be definitely shown to have been undertaken with the avowed purpose of seeing just what would result is not surprising in view of human nature. Enough has been said, however, to make it clear that the Greeks, and the Hippocratics no less than other men of science, were essentially experimentalists and were keen to note and utilize the observations resulting from their practice. Even the one instance of experimentation which one might regard as of a sort to satisfy modern demands is not certainly a true experiment, as is usually assumed. The discovery of the musical concords and intervals, credited to Pythagoreans and doubtless made by use of the monochord, may indeed have been arrived at by stopping the string at definite points to learn what notes would be produced; but it is perhaps more likely that some skillful player or instrument-maker observed and marked on the finger board the intervals and from them deduced the numerical ratios of the musical scale. Nevertheless, the procedure in any case must have been tentative, because on such an instrument as the monochord, the violin, or the guitar, the player must himself "make his note," and, since the Greeks had no means of determining the number of vibrations of the string, the only test of concords and discords or the discrimination of notes was by appeal

SCIENTIFIC METHODS

to the ear. Aristoxenus still operated in that way despite the criticism of Plato,[152] who ridiculed this method, because he demanded an abstract mathematical formula. We must remember that there are still many laws of physics that cannot be demonstrated experimentally with precision, though there are theoretical reasons for supposing them to be correct. In any case, this instance of the musical scale emphasizes the obvious and important fact that the essential factor in the advancement of science was the observation, however it may have been made.

Thus, while it is not fair or in accordance with truth to represent Greek science, or Hippocratic medicine in particular, as relying upon a priori reasoning, or as experimenting only to confirm preconceived notions, one must concede that experimentation had not yet attained either the fundamental importance or the systematic form it has now assumed. The thoroughgoing application of the experimental method is of recent growth. Many experiments were indeed made, but reasoning was for the most part by analogy. We have already pointed out that the limits and the necessary safeguards of reasoning by analogy were not yet sufficiently observed. The point at which all ancient science fell short, however, was in its failure to recognize the infinite complexity of phenomena. The temptation to oversimplify a problem is still very strong; in the early stages of science it was in many cases fatal. One need not confine one's survey to social and psychological experiments to recognize that in many cases the experimenters, for want of an adequate analysis of the subject, have no clear idea of what they are ex-

[152] *Republic*, 530c ff.

perimenting on and that because they cannot isolate or have not isolated the factors involved in a complex their results may be false or misleading. Since the realization of the necessity of isolating the subject, of dealing as it were with a substance chemically pure, comes only by mature experience, it was inevitable that early experimentation should have failed to produce many material results of permanent value. The distinctive service of the experimental method, as applied in modern science, is the discovery and determination of the basic "facts"; the employment of experiment in the testing or confirmation of inferences is probably as old as human intelligence.

VII

MEDICINE AS AN ART

THE HIPPOCRATIC writings are not in general systematic treatises such as one now expects. As has already been pointed out, it is not possible to classify them according to the categories now currently accepted, and often a single work contains matters of very different character. It is, of course, possible to disentangle the interwoven threads of thought and to pursue them singly, and this has been attempted by various writers with satisfactory results. For the purposes of the present discussion it has seemed undesirable to subject the fluid contents of these early writings to the pressure necessary to reduce them to the solid blocks required for a fixed pattern. The Hippocratics were exploring the ground in all directions, but they had not yet divided the fields and fenced them off. In particular, they had not drawn a sharp distinction, even in their thought, between their efforts to create a science of medicine and the urge to perfect their practice in dealing with the concrete problems presented by the twofold task of the physician—to guard against disease and to aid those whom it has assailed. While no consistent attempt has been made in the foregoing account to separate the interests of the Hippocratics, a certain emphasis has fallen on conceptions proper to the development of medicine as a science. In this respect, as has been pointed out, they were children of their age, sharing in good part the views of other contemporary men of science and, doubtless, in part contributing to the common stock of opinion, discoveries, and maturing methods. Yet it is true of Hippocratic medicine, as of all medicine, that it is primarily the application of the science of the day to the practical problems of health and disease. Whatever ambitions individuals, or at times all Hippocratics, may have entertained to found a true science of health, by and large they appear to have been agreed that their immediate task was that of developing and perfecting an art of healing.

As a science proceeds on certain presuppositions and lays down general principles, so an art also is subject to general rules; but an art lays special emphasis on the application of these rules or general conceptions to particular cases, conditions, and circumstances. In considering the Hippocratic art one should, therefore, take account both of the general rules and of their necessary and inevitable special application, which must at times lead to the disregard of recognized rules. The latter aspect of the Hippocratic art would undoubtedly be the most fascinating, were we but in a position to give a detailed account of the procedure of outstanding practitioners in difficult cases. In view of the acknowledged ingenuity and resourcefulness of the Greeks, one readily imagines some extraordinary results achieved, of which there is no record, as well as fatal failures due to desperate expedients.

If the expedients served as deterrents, reflection on them might help to regularize practice; but the results, had they been reported and preserved, might have revolutionized practice. Unfortunately, the record of successes and failures is so inadequate that one is not able to judge how efficient Hippocratic practice actually was. As we have seen, it was recognized that "accidental," or rather unforeseen, results may follow a well-considered course of treatment; for not all Hippocratics shared the optimistic view that medicine, having achieved a sure method, could now dispense with the favors of fortune. Such issues, whether favorable or not, are not to be confused with those arising from a deliberate resort to unusual practice. It was likewise known that in every case it is possible to pursue different courses, some of which will have the same result;[1] consequently, it would fall to the practitioner to make a choice. Nevertheless, he is cautioned not to waver and change his procedure, assuming that it has been reasonably adopted, because the patient does not respond to it according to reasonable expectation—provided, of course, that the doctor has not meanwhile changed his mind.[2] Medicine is defined as a "practice with reason";[3] in other words, as adhering to a recognized procedure while exercising one's intelligence.

The Hippocratics in their practice had in view two objects—the preservation of health and the healing of disease. The state of health was conceived as the true balance of the elements and functions of the body.[4] Essentially

[1] *Epidem.*, VI, vii, 3 (V, 388, Littré).
[2] *Aphorism.*, II, lii (IV, 484, Littré).
[3] *Praecepta*, i (IX, 250, Littré).
[4] Cf. Diocles, frag. 3, Wellmann.

this view is at least as old as Alcmaeon, and it maintained itself throughout. In the absence of many means of physical diagnosis the test of health was naturally the general appearance of the body. It is easy, we are told, to see whether a person is healthy or not if one observes him while he is exercising, stripped, in the gymnasium.[5] The keen and practiced eye of the Greek physician, who was generally either a physical trainer or closely associated with one, thus recognized a state conceived as normal or in accordance with nature.

But, if health could be defined only in general terms, departures from it could be specified by countless indications; for, as Aristotle said, there is only one way to do a thing well, but possible mistakes are numberless.[6] The conception of health remained, therefore, essentially negative—as the absence of disease. In practice Hippocratic medicine was predominantly restorative, seeking to remove the causes of disease and reinstate the patient in the normal condition. It is, however, important to recognize the prominence of prophylaxis in the thought of the Hippocratics. Perhaps the tendency to ignore, or minimize, this aspect is due to the stress laid on the other in the treatise *Regimen in Acute Diseases,* which has generally been credited to Hippocrates himself. The other works of the corpus dealing with questions of diet are quite as much concerned with the preservation of health as with the restoration of the patient.

If one wishes to learn what sort of a regimen was suggested for the maintenance of health, one has only to

[5] *De victu,* I, ii (VI, 470, Littré).
[6] *Nicomachean Ethics,* 1106b.

read the long extract from a treatise of Diocles,[7] preserved by Oribasius. Though it is slightly later in date than the Hippocratics, it nevertheless preserves their spirit and, for the most part, their actual teachings, and its comprehensiveness and orderly arrangement are admirably suited to impress the reader with the sanity and insight of the Greek physician whose aim was to prescribe a regimen calculated to insure health. Dietetics was in fact the very basis of Hippocratic medicine, and the author of *Regimen in Acute Diseases* informs us that many others had written on the subject.[8] The author of *Ancient Medicine* actually regards it as virtually identical with medicine.[9]

Regarding dietaries the Hippocratics were not, naturally, all in agreement, and it would serve no purpose to discuss them in detail or to enumerate the different kinds. The chief requirement was, of course, that the food be digestible or capable of being assimilated. We are told that children's food should be somewhat altered, that of aged persons completely altered, and that of men in their prime, not at all; but this rule would necessarily be subject to exception. Digestion is effected by the internal heat, which is necessary to it.[10] The food is "cooked" in the stomach and intestines;[11] it is even directly spoken of as fuel for the heat, and in certain cases it is suggested that too much may choke and smother the fire.

[7] Frag. 141, Wellmann.
[8] Cap. i (II, 226 f., Littré).
[9] See pp. 106–8.
[10] *De victu salubri*, vii (VI, 82, Littré); and *De victu*, lxxv (VI, 616 f., Littré).
[11] *De morbis*, IV, xliii (VII, 564, Littré).

Growing persons have most innate heat; consequently they require most food, otherwise the body is consumed. Aged persons, however, have but little heat, hence they require little fuel, for it is quenched by large quantities. For this reason also fevers in the aged are not so high, because the body is cold.[12]

The physician could command an adequate variety of foods; indeed, many kinds are mentioned which one would now reject except under extreme necessity.

Next to dietetics, and indeed inseparable from it in the view of the Hippocratics, stood gymnastics as a means of preserving or restoring health. Physical trainers were, of course, employed from early times to supervise the training of athletes for local or national games, as well as for those who daily frequented the gymnasia. Whether they were physicians or not, they must have had or acquired some knowledge of medicine, at least of hygiene. In any case, we know that physicians also visited the gymnasia not only on call, when there was special need, but also as spectators and for the purpose of watching individuals whose condition they wished to observe.[13] In this way there was inevitably brought about a certain interchange of opinion and knowledge and, doubtless in many instances, an actual collaboration, especially in regulating the kind and measure of diet and exercise proper to the individual.[14] There would thus result rules

[12] *Aphorism.*, I, xiv (IV, 466, Littré).
[13] *De victu*, I, ii (VI, 470, Littré).
[14] Plato in various ways indicates the close connection between gymnastics and medicine, though he distinguishes between them, regarding gymnastics as aiming to secure the beauty, medicine the health, of the body. Cf. *Republic*, 403c ff.; *Gorgias*, 452a ff. and 464b ff.; *Sophist*, 228e; and *Politicus*, 295c. *De locis in homine*, xxxv (VI, 326 f., Littré), contrasts them, saying that gymnastics deal with the healthy, medicine with

governing practice not only for those whose condition required to be corrected but also of a more general sort for the preservation of health. Herodicus of Selymbria, who flourished in the last quarter of the fifth century, was reputed to have been the first to formulate such rules. This is hard to believe, except in the sense that he may have been the first to publish a treatise on the subject. From Plato's references to him,[15] one infers that he must have prescribed a regimen calculated to prolong life, even if those who followed it might be said to be only living a lingering death. In Plato's severe judgment such a life was not worth living; but, if one studies the regimen prescribed by Diocles, one recognizes that it too presupposes that he who follows it has no other concern than the care for his health.

Legend said that Herodicus was, after his father, Hippocrates' teacher in medicine, possibly because one of the Hippocratic treatises—*De victu,* Book III [16]—proclaims the author's discovery of the important principle that health depends on the right ratio between nourishment and exercise, while disease results from disproportion between them. Whether or not this formula was then first enunciated, one cannot doubt that in practice it had long been applied by trainers and physicians, as in fact it continued to govern the mode of living prescribed by later writers. Of course, a detailed regimen required further specifications as to kinds and quantities of both

---

the diseased, body; hence, medicine, but not gymnastics, must effect a change in condition.

[15] Especially in the *Republic,* 406a ff. Cf. Euripides, *Supplices,* 1108 ff.
[16] In Littré, VI, 592 and 606 f.

food and exercise. Interesting as the details are, we need not here enlarge upon them.

The Hippocratics naturally laid special stress on the regimen to be followed in acute cases not only because they were those which they were presumably most frequently called upon to treat but because they most often had a fatal issue.[17] If in light or chronic cases an error in judgment might be overlooked or subsequently corrected, acute diseases could not await such tardy amendment.

Life is brief; art is long; but the opportune moment is fleeting. Experiment is risky, and judgment difficult. Hence one must not only oneself do what the situation requires, but the patients also and all who are present. External conditions also must be right.[18]

Such is the situation that confronts the physician in acute cases. We are told that most doctors are bad, and they are likened to bad pilots, who fare well enough in fair weather but suffer shipwreck in a gale.[19] In general the practice, especially in high fevers, was to prescribe ptisan, a light food; but it was recognized that it was necessary to maintain the strength of the patient against the crisis and that it was quite as bad to reduce overmuch his diet as to overfeed him. It is interesting to note that one recognized the benefit that may result in protracted illness from a change in scene, from going abroad to another land.[20] If this suggestion applies to chronic rather than to acute cases, another has special bearing on the acute cases; we read that food, drink, and odors act as restoratives, food requiring

[17] *De victu in acutis*, ii (II, 232, Littré).
[18] *Aphorism.*, I, i (IV, 458, Littré).
[19] *De prisca medicina*, ix (I, 590, Littré).
[20] *Epidem.*, VI, v, 13 (V, 318, Littré).

the longest time and odors the least.[21] Here we have, in effect, the use of smelling salts, though the aromatic substances used are not specified.

Regarding the causes of diseases, the Hippocratics were also not all in agreement.[22] Perhaps the differences were actually less than would at first appear, when *De flatibus* declares that air (gas) is the sole cause of our ills, it is evident that the author thought only of internal medicine. He would hardly have denied the influence of wounds, climate, seasons, epidemics, and unwholesome airs or waters, to which other treatises assign an important role. In general the etiology of the Hippocratics is thoroughly reasonable,[23] the causes assigned being such as a physician today might equally well specify, though he might regard many of them as secondary. Though we know full well from other sources, as also from Hippocratic writings, that superstition was rife among the common people, the physicians were remarkably free from it. Certain visitations were indeed attributed to the gods or to "the divine," but this actually meant very little. The so-called divine or sacred disease (epilepsy) is explained as quite as natural as any other disease.[24] The references to "the divine" as a cause call for most careful study;[25] some of

[21] *De alimento*, 1 (IX, 118, Littré).

[22] *De natura hominis*, ix (VI, 54, Littré), stresses the difference between epidemic diseases and those that befall scattered individuals, the causes of the epidemics being such things as are common to all—for example, infected air—while the causes of the other type must be sought in the mode of living.

[23] See *De natura hominis*, iv (VI, 40, Littré); Philistion, frag. 4, Wellmann; Plato, *Timaeus*, 82 ff.; and Diocles, frag. 3, Wellmann.

[24] *De morbo sacro*, ii (VI, 364, Littré).

[25] See Ludwig Edelstein, "Greek Medicine in Its Relation to Religion and Magic," *Bulletin of the Institute of the History of Medicine*, V

them apparently mean no more than "an act of God," others refer to actions of the elements [26] beyond human control. If any, except those concerned with dreams, ascribe a condition to the direct intervention of the gods, they are extremely few. In other words, there is involved little actual superstition or religion, if by religion one means belief in beings to whom some form of worship is addressed. How the attitude of the Hippocratics in this regard is to be interpreted remains an open question.

In addition to external causes, there were recognized many due to the human constitution. Thus the elementary substances, or the humors, that constitute the body may cause diseases by excess or defect, and the humors especially were thought to be responsible for many ills. They are subject to mixture in various undue proportions, as well as to corruption, in which case they may produce inflammation and suppuration aided by "melting" of the flesh.[27] Most important are noxious mixtures of phlegm or bile with the blood; but heat, cold, moisture, improper diet, and too strenuous exertion may likewise lead to disease. Catarrhal affections appear to have been especially common; one treatise lists seven diseases caused by phlegm.[28] Of the acute diseases, it is now agreed, various kinds of malaria were frequently endemic or epidemic.

It is, perhaps, worth noting that the Hippocratics recog-

(1937), 201 ff.; and Littré, VIII, 527 f. Edelstein's discussion is interesting but not wholly satisfactory.

[26] Cf. *De natura muliebri*, i (VII, 312, Littré). Plato's *Timaeus* is important as throwing light on the ideas: 32d–34b (the generation of the cosmos, the "visible god") and 24b f. Cf. *Politicus*, 295c f.

[27] *De flatibus*, xii (VI, 108, Littré). Cf. Plato, *Timaeus*, 82e–85b.

[28] *De locis in homine*, x (VI, 294 f., Littré).

nized certain diseases as hereditary,[29] though heredity naturally played a minor role in their thought, as was to be expected because of the stress they laid upon the individual constitution. There is a passage in *Ancient Medicine* so significant that it deserves to be quoted at length.

Certain physicians and philosophers assert that nobody can know medicine who is ignorant what man is; he who would treat patients properly must, they say, learn this. But the question they raise is one for philosophy; it is the province of those who, like Empedocles, have written on natural science, what man is from the beginning, how he came into being at the first, and from what elements he was originally constructed. But my view is, first, that all that philosophers or physicians have said or written on natural science no more pertains to medicine than to painting. I hold also that clear knowledge about natural science can be acquired from medicine and from no other source, and that one can attain this knowledge when medicine itself has been properly comprehended, but till then it is quite impossible—I mean to possess this information, what man is, by what causes he is made, and similar points, accurately. This at least I think a physician must know, and be at great pains to know, about natural science, if he is going to perform aught of his duty, what man is in relation to foods and drinks, and to habits generally, and what will be the effects of each on each individual. It is not sufficient to learn simply that cheese is a bad food, as it gives a pain to one who eats a surfeit of it; we must know what the pain is, the reasons for it, and which constituent of man is harmfully affected. For there are many other bad foods and bad drinks, which affect a man in different ways. I would therefore have the point put thus: "Undiluted wine, drunk in large quantity, produces a certain effect upon a man." All who know this would realize

---

[29] *De morbo sacro,* ii (VI, 364, Littré). Cf. *De aere aqua locis,* xiv (II, 58, Littré).

that this is a power of wine, and that wine itself is to blame, and would know through what parts of a man it chiefly exerts this power. Such nicety of knowledge [30] I wish to be attained in all other instances. To take my former example, cheese does not harm all men alike; some can eat their fill of it without the slightest hurt, nay, those it agrees with are wonderfully strengthened thereby.[31] Others come off badly. So the constitutions of these men differ, and the difference lies in the constituent of the body which is hostile to cheese, and is roused and stirred to action under its influence. Those in whom a humor of such a kind is present in greater quantity, and with greater control over the body, naturally suffer more severely. But if cheese were bad for the human constitution without exception, it would have hurt all.[32]

Whether the author of this treatise was a physician or a Sophist makes no difference at all; for it is plain that he expresses the prevailing thought of the Hippocratics. The ideal he proposes for medicine is a high one, still far from being fully attained. What he desires is such a knowledge of foods and of individual constitutions that one may safely prescribe not on the basis of general rules but with special knowledge of the particular patient. Even now the specific actions of few foods and drugs are adequately known, and in the fifth century B.C. the ideal must have appeared impossible of realization.

Nevertheless, in default of such knowledge, the Hippocratics were not wholly at a loss, finding a surrogate, as it were, in their practice of diagnosis. Their object, as we have seen, was to obtain a total unified picture of the patient's condition, not because, as one physician held,

[30] See Chapter II, note 10.
[31] Cf. Aristotle, *Nicomachean Ethics*, 1080b and 1097a.
[32] Cap. xx (I, 620 f., Littré), tr. Jones.

the cause of all diseases was the same, differing only according to the parts affected, but because the whole body was felt to be involved in any ill that befell it. Consequently, their consideration of symptoms was of the most comprehensive sort. In the *Epidemics,* Book I, we have an example:

> The following were the circumstances attending the diseases, from which I formed my judgments, learning from the common nature of all and the particular nature of the individual, from the disease, the patient, the regimen prescribed and the prescriber—for these make a diagnosis more favorable or less; from the constitution, both as a whole and with respect to the parts, of the weather and of each region; from the customs, mode of life, practices and age of each patient; from talk, manner, silence, thoughts, sleep or absence of sleep, the nature and time of dreams, pluckings, scratchings, tears; from the exacerbations, stools, urine, sputa, vomit, the antecedents and consequents of each member in the succession of diseases, and the abscessions to a fatal issue or a crisis, sweat, rigor, chill, cough, sneezes, hiccoughs, breathing, belchings, flatulence, silent or noisy, hemorrhages, and hemorrhoids. From these things we must consider what their consequents also will be.[33]

It is worth noting that in this list of symptoms to be observed there are not a few relating to the state of the patient's mind. In fact, considerable attention was paid to psychic factors;[34] for it was recognized that the physi-

---

[33] Cap. x (II, 668 f., Littré), tr. Jones. Cf. *Epidem.,* III, xvi (III, 100 f., Littré).

[34] There is so much of interest on this topic that one might well devote a chapter to it. The following passages are among those most deserving of attention: *Epidem.,* I, v (II, 636, Littré), I, x (II, 670, Littré), II, iv, 4 (V, 126, Littré), VI, v, 5 (V, 316, Littré), VI, viii, 10 (V, 348, Littré), VI, viii, 17 (V, 350, Littré), and VI, vii, 3 (V, 339, Littré); *De victu,* I, xxxvi (VI, 522, Littré), I, lxi–lxii (VI, 576, Littré),

cian can succeed only with the help of the patient in fighting the disease. In order to enlist and retain his active coöperation, the physician must avoid things that might cause him anxiety—for "worry is a bad disease"[35] —and do anything that he can to win his confidence. An effective means to this end is for the physician to display his knowledge of the normal course of the disease. He is bidden to tell the patient and his friends the previous course of the ailment,[36] to recognize the present stage, to predict what is to come, and to con these matters studiously. He is also asked to have constantly in mind in dealing with ailments two purposes: to be helpful, or at least to do no harm, and to remember that the art of healing involves three factors—the disease, the patient, and the physician. The physician is the servitor of his art, and the patient must combat the disease with the help of the physician. Again we read:

It is best, I think, that a physician practice foresight; for if he knows beforehand and sets forth in the presence of his patients their present state, what has gone before and what is to follow, and states what the patients themselves have failed to observe, he will the more readily be trusted to know the pa-

and III, lxxi (VI, 610, Littré); *De affectionibus,* i (VI, 208, Littré); *De morbis,* I, xxiii (VI, 188, Littré), and IV, xxxix (VII, 558 f., Littré); *De humoribus,* iv (V, 482 f., Littré) and ix (V, 488, Littré); *Prorrhetic,* II, xii (IX, 34, Littré); and *Praecepta,* iv (IX, 254, Littré) and ix (IX, 264, Littré). The treatise *De victu,* especially Book I, presents an interesting and puzzling problem in the view it presents of the "soul" (Ψυχή); see also II, lxi, and IV, lxxxvi.

[35] *De morbis,* II, lxxii (VII, 108, Littré). The reference is specifically to hypochondria, but the word used for "worry" (Φροντίς) is so ordinary that it cannot have been employed as a technical term. Consequently, the sentence must be understood as having a general application.

[36] *Epidem.,* I, v (II, 634 f., Littré).

tients' case, so that men will have the courage to commit themselves to his ministrations; and he will best effect a cure if he foresees what will follow from the present ailments.[37]

The doctor is assumed to be a lover of his kind. "Where there is a love of one's fellowmen, there is also a love of the art";[38] the two are inseparable. When a later physician declared that the practice of medicine was a business like any other, Galen indignantly protested that the great physicians, Hippocrates and Diocles among the rest, were moved by their love of man, not by desire for fame or gain.[39]

One sees that the Hippocratic physician was expected, or at least counseled, to predict the issue of a disease. Though his ability to do so was valued as a potent aid in winning the confidence of his patients and their friends, one can hardly believe that the practice was approved solely or chiefly on that ground. Ambitious as the attempt must appear, it is the natural result of growing confidence in the perfection of medicine. The ability to predict results has always been regarded as the supreme test of a science. We have seen that there were those among the Hippocratics who fondly imagined that medicine was already fully achieved.[40] The treatise *On Decorum* draws an ideal portrait of the man of science,[41] especially the physician and the philosopher, contrasting them with the charlatan, whose character is depicted in the colors familiar

---

[37] *Prognostic*, i (II, 110, Littré).
[38] *Praecepta*, vi (IX, 258, Littré).
[39] *De placitis Hippocratis et Platonis*, V, 751, Kühn.
[40] *De arte*, i (VI, 2, Littré); and *De locis in homine*, xlvi (VI, 342, Littré).
[41] Cap. v (IX, 232, Littré).

from Plato's descriptions of the Sophists. He declares that medicine must be carried into philosophy and philosophy into medicine: the physician is a godlike philosopher. I have elsewhere tried to show that this bold utterance had regard to the ability of the physician to foretell the future.[42] As Diogenes Laërtius says of Democritus: "When he predicted certain events he was held in high esteem, and was henceforth by the multitude accounted worthy of divine honors."[43]

It was not, however, in this spirit that the Hippocratics commonly practiced prognosis. It was obviously done in the interest of the art itself; for, as we note, it was emphasized that the physician can best order the appropriate treatment if he knows the natural issue of the condition that confronts him. Moreover, prognosis was not mere prediction; it was rather knowing without being told. It included knowing the antecedents of the diseased condition and the present symptoms, even when they had failed to be noted by the patient and his friends, as earlier in our discussion we have noted that in a certain case the physician stated that the patient had sometime had epileptic seizures, which his friends had generally ignored or forgotten. Prognosis, thus conceived, was only the total unified picture of the disease in its temporal aspect, knowing its entire course, from antecedents to issue. Having such knowledge, the physician could, of course, be expected to proceed with confidence in the treatment of his patient.

The Hippocratics were, however, well aware that the issue was not always assured: there were many contin-

[42] *The Heroic Age of Science,* pp. 58 ff.   [43] IX, xxxix.

gencies to be reckoned with besides the degree of eager coöperation of the patient. A disease might, seemingly without cause, take one turn or another and accordingly have different possible issues. If such chances marked the limits of the physician's knowledge, they were a challenge to his care and resourcefulness. We have seen how one and another questioned what result might have followed if he had taken another course. Prognosis was not, therefore, a perfected science; it was rather an ideal. Still, it was to be practiced, if for no other reason, because it must lead to closer observation and the foreseeing of possible consequences to be guarded against.

In the last resort the physician must reckon on the help of nature herself. The Hippocratics recognized the inherent recuperative powers of the human organism— "constitutions the healers of diseases"[44]—in minor ills often in themselves sufficient, in acute diseases sometimes the sole reliance of the physician. No wonder, then, that the constitution of the individual patient, the measure of his strength or vitality, his resiliency and responsiveness to treatment, were studied with especial care. Whether the physician believed or not in luck, he must have congratulated himself as well as his patient when he was favored with the help of this powerful ally. The study of the pathological state as such, that characterizes modern medicine, appears to have aroused no particular interest in ancient times. It was rather health, its maintenance or restoration, that wholly engaged the attention of physicians.

Since the Hippocratics had no knowledge of micro-

[44] *Epidem.*, VI, v, 1 (V, 314, Littré).

biology or of germ-diseases their etiology was naturally simplified. Aside from ills that could be attributed to external influences, such as heat or cold, climate, water, tainted air, seasonal changes, or lesions, they recognized others as due to faulty regimen, diet, and physical exertion (too light or too strenuous). In the last resort disease was generally conceived as essentially a state of disturbed balance of the functions and constituent elements of the body. Though the resulting condition might often have been equally well described as due to deficiency of an essential factor, it was more commonly regarded as owing to excess, a humor, say, breaking bounds and overmastering the rest. The cure then consisted in the restoration of the balance by reducing the peccant humor to its proper measure and function. The physician could intervene by inducing evacuation "by the appropriate way,"[45] using emetics, diuretics, or cathartics or by resorting to phlebotomy. In any case, he counted on nature's assistance, recognizing that the peccant matter passed through three stages—crudity, coction, and crisis. Of these stages, the crisis is incomparably the most important, calling for the most careful attention of the physician, because it is in every sense critical. Though it was necessary to maintain the strength of the patient that he might meet the crisis, it was thought wise to reduce somewhat the amount of nourishment just before it arrived.[46]

A crisis did not always arrive; when it did, it decided the turn for the better or the worse. It took various forms, and what immediately followed it required close observa-

[45] *Aphorism.*, I, xxi (IV, 468, Littré).
[46] *Aphorism.*, I, xix (IV, 468, Littré).

tion for fear of a relapse. In connection with the crisis there occurs a term that calls for remark. *Apostasis* seems to have no satisfactory equivalent in modern terminology; for, though it generally signifies an abscess, either simple or metastatic, forming after the subsidence of a high fever, it appears on occasion to refer to a change in the character of a disease itself—for example, from one kind of fever to another. Perhaps we might render it with *metastasis*, if we somewhat enlarge the scope of this term. At any rate, it is significant that the Hippocratics recognized the fact that following a disease attended with high fever, when there has been a definite crisis, there sometimes supervene "after-effects" of a seemingly quite different and unrelated nature.[47]

We have spoken before of the significance that attached to critical days in the eyes of the Hippocratics, and it is not necessary to further enlarge on the subject here. It is unfortunate that the text of *De hebdomadibus* is preserved in so miserable a state; for in cap. xxvii there was obviously given an explanation of the phenomenon that fevers have fixed periods.[48] The attempted explanation was, no doubt, of little or no value, but the recognition of a certain periodicity in their course is of the first importance, because, if the question posed by this fact had been followed up, it might have led much earlier to a deeper and truer understanding of disease.

In view of the character of the Hippocratic treatises, it is obvious that we must expect no single mode of treatment prescribed for the several diseases. Modern physi-

---

[47] Diocles: Aëtius, V, xxix, 1 (Diels, *Doxographi Graeci*, p. 441).
[48] Cf. Plato, *Timaeus*, 89b f.

cians too will be found to differ similarly. Fortunately, the logical principle of the plurality of causes applies in medicine as elsewhere, as we are told in *Epidemics*, "One may give many directions about a single thing, some of which will have the same result." [49] The results to be expected from a course of treatment were known empirically from experience in practice and were, of course, inevitably contingent on many factors and consequently were not invariable. The choice of means lay with the physician, and his success or failure depended in great part on his skill and the range of his experience. The means at his disposal, in foods, exercises, and drugs, were considerable. What a modern physician would think about some of the things prescribed, a layman is not competent to judge; one must bear in mind that the specific actions of foods and drugs, taken singly and in combination, being then, and still, largely unknown, judgment must perforce depend upon experience in treating patients, and then as now there were good physicians and bad physicians. A well-known historian of medicine declares that the greatest value has always been given to the general therapeutic principles of the Hippocratics and that the imperishable fame of Hippocrates rests chiefly on this foundation.[50] Certainly, if one takes into account the limitations of ancient science, it is little short of the marvelous that medicine today should find so much to approve in the practice of these devoted physicians of ancient times.

[49] VI, vii, 3 (V, 338 f., Littré). Cf. *De locis in homine*, xli (VI, 330 f., Littré); and Aristotle, *Topica*, VI, xiii, 12.
[50] Haeser, *Lehrbuch der Geschichte der Medicin*, I, 147.

VIII

CONCLUSION

WHATEVER VALUATION one may place upon Hippocratic medicine, as a whole or in its various details, compared with the medicine of our day its true significance lies in the circumstance that it is the expression of an age of incomparable importance in the intellectual life of the race. We are apt to regard all values as relative, and in a sense that is true; but there is no proportion between one and zero—the relation that virtually subsists between the sixth and fifth centuries B.C. and the earlier ages in respect to the conception and the formulation of scientific ideas. The more one investigates the development of human thought the more obvious it becomes that in this period thinking first became self-conscious, singling out notions and giving them a place and meaning apart from and in contrast to others. Even where the formal definition was not yet achieved, one was already well aware of the scope and connotations of such important terms as nature, matter, force, and quality. Here, then, was laid the very foundation of science, for the distinction between the permanent and the transient, between cause and effect, natural or normal and accidental, health and disease was clearly apprehended: without which a rational view of the world is impossible. In nothing is the thought of this age so set apart from earlier modes of thinking as in its all but complete disregard or rejection of the supernatural in favor of the natural and rational. Daremberg has well said:

With Hippocrates closes the third period of the history of medicine, a period essentially constitutive not only for medicine but also for all the other branches of intellectual culture. It is a decisive period in the destiny of the human race. All the germs of knowledge of the succeeding centuries are contained in it; henceforth everything will proceed from it. It is not a renascence, as in the times of Charlemagne, of Leo X, of Louis XIV; it is the spontaneous movement of the Greek genius, expanding in every direction and creating the best models and the most perfect types in every kind. This primordial fecundity, which has never recurred with equal potency at any time, has never been halted, so, descending from age to age, our nineteenth century is the legitimate offspring of the great age of Pericles. The fifth century of the ancient era is in the intellectual sphere what the first age of the world is in the material.[1]

Another historian of medicine says:

If medicine during more than two thousand years is down to our own day so deeply indebted to the Hippocratics, this is due chiefly to the fact that they for the first time expressed and practiced the eternally true fundamental thought of the art of healing for all times—that its chief object is the practical treatment of the individual patient, that this is to be attained by one's own clinical observation, and that experience is the true teacher of the physician.[2]

---

[1] *Histoire des sciences médicales*, I, 145 f.
[2] Meyer-Steineg, *Geschichte der Medizin*, p. 76.

CONCLUSION

Important as this is, as setting the true course for all who should come in later ages, to our just admiration it is not the sole merit of these bold pioneers. The most competent students of ancient medicine, beginning with Littré and Daremberg, have pointed out a multitude of minute and exact observations recorded in the Hippocratic writings, observations of such nicety that only in most recent times have physicians with incomparably superior equipment repeated and so confirmed them. It is probable that as knowledge advances more and more evidences of the singular insight of the Hippocratics will be found by those who are so fortunate as to know both the achievements of modern science and the ancient record. Here, perhaps more than elsewhere, kindred spirits meet and salute one another across the gulf of intervening ages.

INDEX

Abortion, 38
Acumenus, 59
Acute illness, regimen, 124
Aelian, 110
Aëtius, 42, 45*n*; quoted, 87
Aftereffects, of treatment, 37; of crisis, 135
Air, 19, 20, 92; proved a corporeal substance, 50; controlling agent of the body, 52, 54, 125; contained in water, 111
Alcmaeon, 42–49, 100, 120; Pythagorean influence on, 43, 45; as an intelligent physician and man of science, 43; his date and connections, 43; as an example of the ideals and methods of the medical profession, 44
Alexander Polyhistor, 43
"All things together," theory, 49
Analogies, assumed, 77; from biology, 83; from physics, 83, 85, 96; having to do with fundamental conceptions of Hippocratics, 86; physiological, 95
Analogy, reasoning by, 76, 115; reasoning as result of experimentation, 96
Anatomy, earliest treatise on, 29; systematic, 53; limited knowledge of, 58
Anaxagoras, 10, 13, 52, 92, 100, 111; as physician and scientist, 49–51

Anaximander, 16, 47, 89
"Anaximander's Book . . ." (Heidel), 17*n*
Anaximenes, 19, 52, 112
Ancient Medicine, xiv, 83, 121; excerpts, 81, 106, 127
Animals, dissection of, 47, 51, 53, 58; misconceptions arising from dissection, 78; diseases explained by observations on, 84
Antiphon, 44
Antisthenes, 3
Aphorism, excerpts, 122, 124
Apollo, 27
Apology of Socrates (Plato), 40
Apostasis, 135
Archytas, 95
Aristippus of Cyrene, 3
Aristophanes, 104
Aristotle, vii, ix, 5, 6, 13, 16, 17, 19, 29, 52, 53, 72, 109, 120; regard for greatness of Hippocrates, xiii, 14; esteem for physicians, xiv; Berlin Academy edition, xv; quoted, 21, 22, 32, 33, 92; indebted to medical tradition for his first philosophy, 41 f.; information about Alcmaeon, 42–46 *passim;* on particular *vs.* general, 76; physiological analogies, 96; conclusions and experiments, 97; theory re sea water, 110; on respiration in water, 111
Aristoxenus, 115

INDEX

Art, medicine as an, 31, 117–36; rules and their application, 118
Asclepius, god, 2, 27
Astronomy, 16, 44
Athens, plague at, 61, 62
Athletes, observation of, 77, 122
Atomists, 45
Attraction, caused by heat, 88; process of, 90
Aulus Gellius, 106

Babe, development of, 83, 87
Bacon, Francis, opinions about Aristotle, 97
Bacon, Roger, 99
Berlin Academy, edition of Aristotle, xv
Biology, analogies from, 83
Body, knowledge of, linked with knowledge of universal nature, vii, xi, 11, 13, 22, 127; elements composing, 47, 54; cure begins with soul, 53; affects entire organism, 54, 55; recuperative powers, 59, 133; stress laid upon individual constitution, 127
Boyle, Robert, 99
Brain, investigation of, 48
Breathing a form of nutrition, 80, 81; see also Respiration
Bro[n]tinus, 44n

Capacities requisite to successful practice, 73
Capillarity, 94, 113
Casebooks, 60, 62
Cause, 63, 68; knowledge of, 58; opinions concerning, 125 ff.; principle of plurality of, 136
Celsus, 20
Chalcidius, 47
Chance, 109, 133
Change in scene, 124
Charlatans, 30, 131

Charms, Thracian, 53
Christian saints of healing, 1
Cicero, 28
Circular displacement, 93
Circulation, from organ to organ, 50; of body fluids, 93
Clans and guilds, 27
Clouds (Aristophanes), 104
Cnidian school of medicine, 2, 23, 67; distinction between school of Cos and, 83
Coan praenotions, illustrations from, 70
Coan school of medicine, 2, 23, 24, 67; distinction between Cnidian school and, 83
Code, medical, 27
Cold, and heat, 86, 93, 112; influence upon veins, 89
Complexity of phenomena, failure to recognize, 20, 115
Conception, 92
Constitutions, compared with medical treatises, 33
Consultation, 36
Contraries, 43n, 46
Cosmas, 1
Cosmology, temperature, 86, 87
Coughing, epidemic of, 61
Court physician, 26, 27
Crisis, 124, 134 f.; doctrine of, 68
Critias (Plato), 41
Culture-gods and heroes, 108
Cupping instruments, 82
Curative force of body, 59, 133

Damian, 1
Daremberg, Charles-Victor, 139; quoted, 138
De affectionibus, 64n; excerpt, 109n
De arte, 65, 75; authorship, 74; excerpt, 74
De articulis, 77; cited, 36; excerpt, 37

INDEX

De caelo (Aristotle), 96
De carnibus, 89; excerpt, 90
De flatibus, 52, 54, 125
De hebdomadibus, 135
De humoribus, excerpt, 65
De liquidorum usu, 71
Delirium, 70
Democedes, 27
Democritus, 20, 109, 110, 111, 132
De morbis, excerpts, 106, 111
De nutrimento, 53, 54
De respiratione (Aristotle), excerpt, 111
De victu, 53, 54, 85, 90, 123
Dewey, John, xv
Diagnosis, ix, 55, 61, 64, 127, 128; anatomical tests, 66; regarded as prognosis, 68
Diels, Hermann, xv
Diet, test of digestibility, 66; specific action of foods, 81, 127, 128; the basis of medicine, 121; ratio between nourishment and exercise, 123; in acute cases, 124
Dietaries, chief requirements, 121
Digestion, 121; test, 66
Diocles, xv, 29, 38*n*, 53, 85, 131; regimen to insure health, 121, 123
Diodorus Siculus, quoted, 100
Diogenes Laërtius, on Democritus, 132
Diogenes of Apollonia, 19, 44, 91, 111; influence of, 51 f.; views, 52; explanation of Nile floods, 94
Diogenes the Cynic, xiv; quoted, xv
Displacement of substance, 93
Dissection of animals, *see* Animals
Divine, the, as cause of disease, 125
Doctors, *see* Medical profession
Dogmatics, 2
Doxographic tradition, 42, 52

Drink, goes to lungs, 105; and food, 106
Dropsy, 84
Dryden, John, quoted, 8*n*

Earth, 19, 20
Education, 28
Egypt, floods, 94, 101; alluvial soil, 101; age, 102
Eleatics, 42
Elements, the four, 19, 20; of the body, 46 f., 54; range in cosmology, 86
Empedocles, 20, 47, 92, 95, 100, 127; four elements of, 19, 21; as physician and scientist, 49, 50; theories of, 78, 87, 88, 90
Empirics, 2, 72
Environment, dependence of health and disease upon, 23, 63
Epicharmus, 75
Epicurus, 81
Epidemics, 61; causes, 125*n*
Epidemics, 55, 61, 67, 71, 72, 136; excerpt, 129
Epilepsy, 84, 125, 132
Erasistratus, 50, 53, 93, 106
Eryximachus, 59
Eudemus, 42
"Evacuated, pursuit of the," 93
Evaporation, 111 ff.
Evidence on which conclusions based, not disclosed, 98
Evolution, idea dimly caught, x
Exercise, 122, 123
Experience, knowledge based upon, 59, 60
Experimentation, observations derived from, 47, 50, 53, 100–116; analogical reasoning as result of, 96; Aristotle's concern with, 97; evidence not disclosed, 98; value of Hippocratic method, 100; pro-

INDEX

Experimentation (*Continued*)
cedure in discovery of musical scale, 114

Facies Hippocratica, 67
"Father of Medicine," xiii
Fees, 38n
Fetus, 83, 87
Fevers, 87, 135
Fire, 19, 20
Fish, respiration, 110
Flattery, arts of, 10
Floods of the Nile explained, 94, 101
Fluids of body, *see* Humors
Food, *see* Diet
Foresight, 68, 130, 131
Fragmente der Vorsokratiker, Die (Diels), xv
Fragmentsammlung der griechischen Aerzte (Wellmann), xv

Galen, 2, 4, 23, 28, 64n, 131
Generalization, process of, 71, 73, 75–77; passage from observation of particulars to, 76, 98
Geschichte der Medizin (Meyer-Steineg), excerpt, 138
Gods of healing, 27
Gomperz, Theodor, 74
Gorgias, the rhetorician, 35
Gorgias (Plato), 80, 110
Greeks, lay foundations of science, v, vi; link between science and philosophy, vi, 16; intelligence and imagination, vii; link knowledge of the body with knowledge of universal nature, vii, xi, 11, 13, 22; questions raised by, viii; the first scientific physicians, ix; handicapped by static natural philosophy, x; intellectual awakening during sixth and fifth centuries B.C., 15, 137 f.; literature didactic, 69
Guilds and clans, 27
Gymnastic trainers, 77, 120, 122
Gynecology, 91

Haeser, Heinrich, quoted, 39, 60
Healing, Christian saints of, 1; gods of, 27; and health preservation, as double objective, 119
Health, relation to environment, 23, 63; conception and preservation of, 119, 120; tests, 120; regimen for maintenance of, 120, 123 f.
Heat, innate, 50, 87 f., 93, 121; and cold, 86, 93, 112; in cosmology, 86, 87; attraction caused by, 88, 92; digestion effected by, 121
Hecataeus of Miletus, 103
Heidel, William Arthur, studies of early Greek period, v; writings, v, 17, 18n, 100n
Hellebore, 31
Heraclitus, 44, 46, 47, 53, 110
Heredity, 127
Herodicus of Selymbria, 9, 35, 123
Herodotus, 27; quoted, 101, 102; importance as a witness, 101
Heroic Age of Science, The (Heidel), v; excerpt, 100
Herophilus, 53
Hesiod, 17
Hidden ailments and conditions, 65, 75
Hippocrates, called Father of Medicine, xiii; Aristotle's regard for greatness of, xiii, 14; slight knowledge of, 1, 2; status: invoked as saint, 1; ancestry, dates, 2; invoked by all schools of medicine, 2, 4; question of his views and writings, 3, 7, 8, 14; Plato's knowledge of, 3, 4, 8–14 *passim;* period in which he bore

INDEX

leading part, 4; moved only by love of man, 38n, 131; *Regimen in Acute Diseases* accredited to, 120, 121; teacher of, 123; foundation of fame, 136

Hippocratic oath, formulation of, 27 f., 38

Hippocratics, *see* Medical profession

Hippocratic writings, system of interpretations, vii; by many authors, vii, 4, 24, 32; editions cited, xv; similarities in knowledge and conceptions, 5, 18; Plato's views in accord with, 9; value to student of ancient philosophy and science, 17; conception of medicine, 21, 22; recourse to, a common practice, 32-34; not systematic, difficult to disentangle and arrange, 57, 117; recording of observations, 60; literary standards, 69; method of procedure, 70; comparisons in forms of similies and metaphors, 79 f.

Histoire des sciences médicales (Daremberg), excerpt, 138

History of the Inductive Sciences (Whewell), v

Homer, 16

Homologies, 78

Horror vacui, 93

Household remedies, collection of, 64n

Humors, circulation, 50, 93; attraction of, 51; theory of the four, 54; pathology, 58, 126; power an intensity of, 81; organs conceived as reservoirs of, 94

Hypochondria, 130n

Iamblichus, xv
Identity, 76, 78
Ilberg, Johannes, quoted, 24

Immortality of soul, 44, 45

Individual patient, Hippocratics chiefly concerned with, 63, 76; stress laid upon individual constitution, 127; *see also* Body

Individuation, principle of, 20n

Induction, 72

Inference, 72, 75, 76

Innate heat, *see* Heat

Instruction, individual, 28

Intellectual life of Greece, incomparable importance of age of, 15, 137 f.; ancient medicine an expression of, 137

Intellectual outlook of physicians, 37

Intellectual process described, 73

Intelligence, use of, the essential contribution of Greeks, ix; distinction between sense perception and, 48

Investigation, theory undeveloped, 73; by the light of facts, 75; *see also* Experimentation

Ion of Chios, 109n

Isolation of subject, 116

Jesus Christ, 3
Josiah Macy, Jr. Foundation, v, xv

Kast, Ludwig, xv; foreword, v-xi
Knowledge, interest in the advancement of, 108; display of, 130, 131

Laws (Plato), excerpt, 36
Legislation, written: compared with medical treatises, 33
Leucippus, 52, 93
Life of Pythagoras (Porphyry), 43
Lips, compressed, 82
Liquid, finds way into lungs, 105
Literature, didactic character of Greeks, 69; does not disclose full

Literature (*Continued*)
  account of evidence and studies, 98; *see also* Hippocratic writings
Littré, Émile, xv, 5, 29, 61, 83, 139
Logic, formal or deductive, 72; empirical, 73
Love, of physician for his kind, 38*n*, 131; the two kinds, 59
Lucretius, 49
Lungs, liquid reaches, 105

Machaon, 108
Macy, Josiah, Jr., Foundation, v, xv
Magnetism, phenomena of, 90
Maspero, Gaston Camille Charles, quoted, 98
Mathematicians, views of, 44, 45
Matter, Empedocles' classification, 49
Medical profession, belief that patient must be understood as part of universal nature, vii, xi, 11, 13, 22, 127; scientific spirit, viii, ix, 17, 31, 37; Plato's opinion of, xiv, 9, 30, 31, 34 ff.; the product of the thought of the age, 18, 118, 137; theories about what things are made of, 19; long and honorable career, 26; court physicians, 26, 27; clans and guilds, 27; code governing conduct, 27; Hippocratic oath, 27 f., 38; instruction, 28 f., 32; the doctor's calling, 29, 36, 39, 55; recourse to written treatises, 32; intellectual outlook, 37; moral requisites, 38; love and spirituality, 39, 60, 131; some outstanding scientists, 40–56; not yet a closed corporation, 40; scientific methods, 57–116; achievements notable but new facts not to be gleaned from their meager knowledge, 57; freedom from superstition, 62, 125, 126, 138; chiefly concerned with individual patient, 63, 76; aimed at a total unified picture, 67; foresight and prognosis, 68, 70, 130, 131, 132 f.; physical trainers, 77, 120, 122; efforts to coördinate what they learned, 79; preservation of health, and healing, their double objective, 119; successes and failures impossible to gauge, 119; ideal portrait of physician, 131; chief reasons for modern valuation of, and indebtedness to, 136, 138; *see also* Hippocrates; Scientists
Medicine, link with philosophy, vi, 17, 20, 37, 132; task of focusing all knowledge upon problem of man's welfare, vii, xi; Hippocratics aimed to make scientific, viii; Hippocratic period, 5; defined, 6, 119; public speaking procedure compared with that of, 10; as conceived by Hippocratic writers, 21, 22; not an exact science, 30; as an art, 31, 117–36; comparison between treatises or written legislation, 33; Aristotle's indebtedness to medical tradition, 41; unduly speculative and dogmatic, 69; predominantly restorative, 120; *see also* Science
Medicine, schools of: Hippocrates claimed and invoked by nearly all, 2, 4; Cnidian, 2, 23, 67, 83; Coan, 2, 23, 24, 67, 83; Sicilian, 9, 49; differences revealed in Hippocratic writings, 23 f.; of Miletus, 52; philosophy of Heraclitus, 53
Melissus, 42
Membranes, formation of, 88

INDEX

Menodotus, 72
Menon, 19, 42
Mental state, 129
Metals, 91
Metaphors and similies, comparison in the forms of, 79
Meteorologica (Aristotle), 96
Meyer-Steineg, quoted, 138
Miletus, school of, 52
Monistic doctrines, 54
Moral requisites, physicians', 38
Mother, heat derived from, 87
Musical scale, deduction of numerical ratios, 114
Myson, 75

Natural science, *see* Science
Nature, knowledge of universal, linked with knowledge of body, vii, xi, 11, 13, 22, 127; recuperative powers, 59, 133
Necessity the mother of invention, 108
Nicomachean Ethics (Aristotle), excerpt, 32
Nile floods, explained, 94, 101
Novum organum (Bacon), 97
Nutrients, 80; *see also* Diet
Nutrition, breathing a form of, 80, 81

Observation, derived from experiment, 47, 50, 53, 100–116; and record, 60–62; passage from, to generalization, 76, 93
Odyssey, excerpt, 26
Œuvres complètes d'Hippocrate (Littré), xv
On Decorum, 131
On Epilepsy, 84
On Internal Diseases, 84
On Nature, 41
On the Art, see *De arte*
On the Heart, excerpt, 105

Opposites, 43n, 46
Oratory, procedure compared with that of medicine, 10
Oribasius, 121

Parmenides, 42
Particular *vs.* the general, 76
Pericles, 10, 12
Periodicity, perceived by Greeks, 68; of fevers, 135
Phaedrus (Plato), 10
Pharmakitis, 64n
Philosopher, earliest, 16
Philosophy, link with science and medicine, vi, 16, 17, 20, 37, 132; idea of evolution lacking, x; concern of, 15
Physical elements (roots), conception of, 49
Physical trainers, 77, 120, 122
Physician, 38
Physicians, *see* Medical profession
Physics, analogies from, 83, 85, 96
Physiology, human: laws of, only special forms of universal laws, 23; little known, 58
Plague at Athens, 61, 62
Plato, ix, xiii, 3, 6, 16, 40, 53, 59, 72, 80, 97, 106, 109, 110, 115, 132; opinion of doctors, xiv, 9, 30, 31, 34 ff.; edition of Stephanus, xv; knowledge of Hippocrates and of medicine, 3, 4, 8–14 *passim;* discussion of respective merits of rule by statesman and under written code, 33; quoted, 35; philosophy and interests, 41; connection between gymnastics and medicine, indicated, 122n; judgment on prolonging life, 123
Plutarch, 51, 106, 109n
Pneuma doctrine, 52
Podaleirius, 108

INDEX

Polar expressions, 86
Politics (Aristotle), 33
Polybus, 64*n*
Porphyry, 43
Powers and structures, 81
Praxagoras, 66
Prediction, 131, 132
Preservation of health, 119
Problems (pseudo-Aristotelian), 44
Prognosis, 68, 70; practice of, 130, 132 f.
Prognostic, 71; excerpt, 131
Prorrhetic, illustrations from, 70
Protagoras, 74, 109
Psychic factors, 129
Public speaking, procedure compared with that of medicine, 10
Pulse, 66
Putrefaction, 88
Pythagoras, 1, 20; Porphyry's *Life of*, 43
Pythagoreans, regard for art of medicine, xv; relation of Alcmaeon to, 43, 45; scheme of ten pairs of contraries, 43*n*, 46; other notions, 45, 81; discovery of muscial concords and intervals, 114

Reason, themes of unreason and, 10, 13; analyzed, 73; *see also* Intelligence
Reasoning by analogy, 76, 115; result of experimentation, 96
Recording of observations, 60–62
Recuperative powers of organism, 59, 133
Regimen for maintenance of health, 120, 123 f.
Regimen in Acute Diseases (Hippocrates?), 120, 121
Religion, origin, 16
Republic (Plato), 8, 41, 80

Respiration, 50, 80, 93; in water, 110; evaporation regarded as, 112
Restoratives, 124
Roots (physical elements), conception of, 49

Sack of Troy, 108
Salt water, 110, 113
Savors, perception of, 91
Scaevola, 28
Schools of medicine, *see* Medicine, schools of
Science, Greeks lay foundations of, v, vi, ix, 137; link with philosophy, vi, 16, 20; current outlook reflected by medicine, 6; concern of philosophy and, 15; Greeks concerned with whole range of, 16; beginning of specialization, 17; concern with what things are made of, 19; failure to recognize complexity of phenomena, 20, 115; conception of medicine as, 21, 37; scientific methods of physicians, 57–116; *see also* Medicine
Scientific terminology and practice, 75
Scientists, outstanding, 40–56; Aristotle, and Plato, 41; Alcmaeon, 42–49; Empedocles, 49, 50; Anaxagoras, 49–51; Diogenes of Apollonia, 51–53; ideal portrait of man of science, 131; *see also* Medical profession; *also entries under men listed*, *e.g.*, Aristotle
Seneca, quoted, 94
Sense organs, investigation of, 48
Sicilian school of medicine, 9, 49
Similarities, generalization proceeds upon assumption of, 76; noting of, 80

INDEX 149

Similies and metaphors, comparison in the forms of, 79
Simples, physicians' preference, 20n
Simplicius, 52
Skeptics, 2, 72
Slaves, 35
Smelling salts, 125
Socrates, ix, 1, 3, 5, 10, 40, 41, 53n, 72, 80, 86, 104, 110
Sophocles, 109n
Soul, immortality, 44, 45; cure of body begins with, 53
Speculation, 69
Spiritual basis of treatment, 39, 60, 131
Spontaneous, the, 109n
Stephanus, edition of Plato, xv
Structures and powers, 81
Substances of which things are made, 19
Suction, 90, 92, 93
Superstition, freedom from, 62, 125 126, 138
Surface tension, 94
Surgery, 57
Symptoms, study of, 62, 64, 129; see also Diagnosis

Temperature, in cosmology, 86, 87; see also Heat
Terminology, scientific, 75
Tests, 66, 120
Textbooks, 29
Thales, 44
Theophrastus, 17, 41, 42, 45n, 48, 52, 110
Therapeutic principles, value placed upon, 136

Thracians, medical theory, 53
Thucydides, 61, 62
Timaeus (Plato), 9, 17, 41
Trainers, physical, 77, 120, 122
Treatises, recourse to written, 32–34; comparison between written legislation or constitutions and, 33; see also Hippocratic writings
Treatment, rarely mentioned in casebooks, 61

Universal laws, laws of human existence as forms of, vii, xi, 11, 13, 22, 127

Vacua in body, 91 ff.
Valetudinarianism, 9
Veins, 53, 88
Visible and known, inference from, 75
Vivisection, 47

Water, one of elements, 19, 20; liquids analogous to, 91; effect of surface tension upon, 94; salt, 110, 113; air content, 111; evaporation, 111; weights, 113
Water clock, 50, 87
Wellmann, Max, xv
Whewell, William, v, 97
Worry, 130

Xenophanes, 108
Xenophon, 80

Zeno, 42

Bei Fragen zur Produktsicherheit wenden Sie sich bitte an:
If you have any questions regarding product safety,
please contact:

Walter de Gruyter GmbH
Genthiner Straße 13
10785 Berlin
productsafety@degruyterbrill.com